MW00788575

MASTER YOUR CORE

A Science-Based Guide to Achieve
Peak Performance and Resilience to Injury

Dr. Bohdanna Zazulak

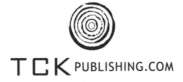

TCK PUBLISHING.COM

Copyright © 2021 by Dr. Bohdanna Zazulak.

All Rights Reserved.

No part of this publication may be reproduced, distributed, or trans-mitted in any form or by any means, including photocopying, record-ing, or other electronic or mechanical methods, or by any information storage and retrieval system without the prior written permission of the publisher, except in the case of very brief quotations embodied in critical reviews and certain other noncommercial uses permitted by copyright law.

ISBN: **978-1-63161-116-2**

Sign up for Bohdanna Zazulak's newsletter at
www.doczaz.com/newsletter

Published by TCK Publishing
www.TCKpublishing.com

Get discounts and special deals on our best selling books at
www.TCKpublishing.com/bookdeals

Check out additional discounts for bulk orders at
www.TCKpublishing.com/bulk-book-orders

Table of Contents

Medical Disclaimer

This book contains information and guidelines related to health, wellness, and injury prevention. All materials, including text, graphics, and images are for informational purposes only and are not a substitute for medical diagnosis, advice, or treatment. All readers should seek expert medical care, advice, and guidance before embarking on any exercise program, and for all general or specific health issues. The author and the publisher disclaim any liability, loss, or risk (personal or otherwise) which is incurred as a consequence, either directly or indirectly, of the use or application of any of the material in this publication.

To Daria and Walter Zazulak
who gave life and soul to the seed of my core.
May everyone be so nurtured to flourish!

Foreword

When I first met Dr. Zazulak two decades ago, she was presenting her research on injury disparities between the sexes at the annual American Physical Therapy Association Conference in Nashville, Tennessee. I was impressed not only by her vast understanding of sports biomechanics, but also her theoretical reasoning and passion for protecting lives from devastating injuries. I was even more struck by her remarkable ability to think outside the box, recognize the big picture, and provide actionable advice.

Modern scientific study tends to cause researchers to oversimplify things: because of reductionism and hyperspecialization, researchers and clinicians often see only the trees but not the forest. Science is not merely the collection of data and facts; it involves a method of investigation that fosters the discovery of novel knowledge (and a way to use that knowledge to get better results in the real world). A closed mind of blind certainty has no room for new knowledge, whereas an open mind is the window to the universe. Dr. Zazulak's insightful holistic thinking starts with an open mind, and is what inspired our award-winning research establishing the importance of the core for overall health and injury prevention.

In addition to her prestigious career and her invaluable contributions to evidence-based science, I am most impressed with Dr. Zazulak's intellectual curiosity, creative insight, compassion, and positive outlook, which is evident in the way she approaches every aspect of life. This makes her an asset to every single one of her patients, colleagues, and readers, as well as the future direction of health and injury prevention.

Over the years, we have continued our collaborative efforts with national and international scientists and healthcare professionals. We have published extensive peer-reviewed manuscripts and books, and have presented many national and international symposia to share our knowledge of core health and injury prevention.

Recently, the coronavirus pandemic has drawn attention to the darkness looming over global health and the shortcomings of our current healthcare systems. People throughout the world are finally recognizing that most diseases and premature deaths are preventable with lifestyle modification, and are seeking guidelines to add more years to life, and more life to the years they have.

Dr. Zazulak's voice will carry the farthest over the sea of popular health and exercise recommendations, as this program is based on science. Science will always prevail over empty promises of unfounded fitness crazes, which too often serve the dangerous injustice of causing injuries instead of preventing them. Understanding the science motivates us to make substantial investments and improvements in our own health, and the health of those around us. *Master Your Core* will guide you with a proactive strategy to discover and develop the magical pearl of the core, to illuminate and fortify your fitness, mindset, spirit, and wellbeing from within you.

—Dr. Timothy Hewett, world-renowned injury prevention expert

Introduction

"Health is a state of complete harmony of the body, mind, and spirit.
When one is free from physical disabilities and mental distractions,
the gates of the soul open."
—B.K.S. Iyengar

Terrell Davis won the Super Bowl MVP title after leading the Denver Broncos to victory with three rushing touchdowns on January 25, 1998. As one of the best running backs in the NFL, his career was on track to keep rising. But when he tore his anterior cruciate ligament (ACL) during the 1999 season, all his dreams were suddenly crushed. The ACL, a crucial stabilizer of the knee, is a tissue that connects the thigh bone with the shin bone. After injuring this ligament, Terrell was never again able to play at the same level, despite undergoing multiple surgeries, physical therapy, and the best sports rehabilitation money can buy. He retired from the NFL in 2002.

What could this man have achieved had he not suffered such an unfortunate injury? How many rushing records could he have broken in the NFL? How many more Super Bowls could he have helped his team win? When someone suffers a devastating injury like that, they can sometimes recover. Surgery and physical therapy can do great things, but not every injury can be perfectly fixed or healed. Sometimes recovery is only partial, and that means people like Terrell Davis can't walk, run, or move like they could before the injury occurred.

But for every story like Terrell Davis's, there are four to six times more stories of women who suffer the same life-changing ACL injuries (including Megan Rapinoe, Rebecca Lobo, Lindsay Vonn, Misty May-Trainer, and millions more). That's because women suffer far more of these injuries than men. Even though the injuries of male athletes attract most of the media headlines in sports, there are millions of untold stories of female athletes whose lives and careers have been harmed because of their injuries.

There are more than one hundred thousand ACL surgeries performed every year, and that's just for one kind of injury. We're talking about millions of women, men, children, and teenagers every year who suffer injuries they may never fully recover from, even if they all had

1

access to the very best medical care possible. The good news is that many of these injuries are completely preventable, and we can save millions of people from needless suffering once we stop bad training habits and start implementing the key lessons from modern research on proper training and injury prevention.

The Impact of Injuries

"There is no ghost so difficult to lay as the ghost of an injury."
—Alexander Smith

The magnitude of pain, suffering, and revenue loss from these injuries is staggering. Terrell Davis lost millions of dollars in potential earnings, and his dream career was cut short. Granted, not everyone who gets injured misses out on multi-million-dollar opportunities, but the costs are enormous when you consider the sheer number of people who suffer injuries that are often preventable. As many as one out of every two professional and amateur athletes who get injured are no longer able to play the sports they love. Millions of people lose their jobs because they can no longer move their bodies in the same way. Each year, over 50 million adults report a total of over 500 million days of work lost due to injuries, with women reporting more workdays lost than men.

How did we get here? How is it possible that despite millions spent in sports therapy, training, and the best medical care available, young, healthy athletes of all levels continue to be plagued by life-changing injuries from which many never recover? Time and time again, the answer lies at the core. Unfortunately, the commercialization and misappropriation of the term "core stability" too often preaches the importance of never-ending sit-ups, only to lead even the most "fit" to a life of pain and injury. We'd all love to have six-pack abs, but that's not what will escort you to your best, injury-free life. This book will show you how to focus on your core as a powerhouse of physical, emotional, and spiritual power, so you can give it the care it deserves.

You'll also learn how to train your mind and body to be less susceptible to these kinds of life-changing injuries. In the process, you'll receive valuable tips for dramatically improving your performance in all activities and enhancing your overall health and wellbeing by awakening your core, the anatomical center of your body.

I have dedicated my career, beginning with my undergraduate research thirty years ago, to an impassioned quest for answers regarding injury rate disparities between the sexes. I wanted to find out why so many women were being injured, and learn what could be done to prevent injuries for all and help the injured heal from that pain.

My lifelong pursuit of these answers led me to my award-winning research determining that core instability is directly related to injury. We now know that core training significantly lowers injury rates in both women and men, as demonstrated in successful injury prevention programs around the world.

I have published extensively on this important topic and presented my research to our national and international medical community. Working as a Doctor of Physical Therapy at Yale for many years, I have treated countless patients of all ages whose lives might have taken a different course had they known in advance how to empower their cores to prevent injury and pain.

Google receives over one billion health-related questions each day. Accessing health information has never been easier, yet the challenge is determining what will help you and what will hurt you. This book will teach you the current evidence-based science of core stability and injury prevention that is valid and reliable, presented in a language that anyone can understand. You'll also get a step-by-step guide for empowering your core. This will lead to countless benefits, including fewer injuries, less pain, and better overall health, and all of it is backed by solid research that many of my esteemed colleagues and I have conducted.

Why Core Health Is Important

"Grant me the serenity to accept the things I cannot change, the courage to change the things I can, and the wisdom to know the difference."
—Reinhold Niebuhr

Your chance of sustaining any type of injury is linked to your unique physical, psychological, and emotional make-up, as well as factors from the world around you.

The list of researched predictors of injury and illness is extensive, and includes: having a previous injury (history tends to repeat); anatomy and size (the bigger you are, the harder you fall); pain (especially for those who follow the erroneous "no pain, no gain" philosophy); hormonal fluctuations; insufficient sleep; fatigue; inadequate nutrition; poor self-care; poor cardiovascular health; genetic predisposition; emotional stress; competitive and aggressive personality; psychological unpreparedness; fear of injury; extent of sports practice and participation; excessive training; lack of flexibility; weakness; faulty biomechanics; diminished balance; and impaired core stability, which is a key element of successful prevention programs.

Risk of injury also depends on environmental variables such as equipment, ground surfaces, and safety hazards that may not be within your control. In other words, there are a lot of ways to be injured, and some factors can't be avoided. Regardless of any protective equipment you wear, how cautious you try to be, or how lucky you get, you cannot prevent all injuries or illnesses. Yet, the healthier your core is, the lower your risk.

If you think of your body as a car, one aspect of your core may be represented by shock absorbers. Most people worry about having flashy red paint or fine leather seats in their cars, because these are the things that other people can see; but if the shock absorbers aren't resilient and responsive, the car will break down fast. The human body must be able to absorb shocks and impacts from 360 degrees. Just as we preoccupy ourselves with the style and speed of our cars, we place most of our focus on making our bodies stronger, faster, or more "beach-ready." But if you only work on strength and speed, you'll be in more danger and even more likely to suffer injuries, simply because you don't have resilient and responsive shock absorbers to protect you from the extra forces of the added strength and speed.

This book will teach you how to take the driver's seat and reclaim control of your core to dramatically reduce your risk of injury in sports and everyday life using proven and effective strategies. I invite you to embark on your own journey to core empowerment for a healthy life with a sculpted body that works the way you need and want it to. You'll be armed with the knowledge and tools you need to reprogram your mind and core to achieve holistic health and wellness, the best-known way to reduce injuries and relieve pain. As Benjamin Franklin said, "An ounce of prevention is worth a pound of cure."

How Empowering Your Core Prevents Injuries

"It is never too late to be who you might have been."
—George Eliot

To help you understand the importance of proper core training, I'll walk you through expert analysis of core health. We'll address core stability from a holistic perspective, which includes your body, mind, and spirit, because research shows these three areas are crucial for developing resilience to injuries. Education is the key to lasting empowerment and injury prevention, and after reading this book you'll know exactly what you need to do to prevent injuries.

Doing core exercises is great, but if you don't understand why the core is so important and how you can improve your core health beyond physical exercise, you won't reach your full potential. My purpose in writing this book is to share the fundamental concepts of what I have learned through my extensive research and three decades of clinical experience as a physical therapist at Yale.

You will learn to reduce your risk of physical problems, such as overuse injuries, pelvic floor dysfunction, broken bones, and back, shoulder, knee, and foot injuries, to name just a few benefits of properly training your core. If you follow the training in this book, you'll be less likely to end up in the ER with a torn ACL, broken bone, or severe muscle spasms, saving you an enormous amount of pain, money, and months (or even years) of rehabilitation. Devastating injuries like a torn ACL increase risk of arthritis by at least 50 percent, double the likelihood of requiring a knee replacement, and set off a cascade of damaging physical and psychological effects on the body that we are just beginning to understand. I wouldn't wish such an injury on my worst enemy, and I don't want you to suffer from one either. I created this book to help you and millions of others understand this critical information so you don't have to go through that kind of needless pain and suffering.

There are several books out there purporting to teach core stability, yet none of the books I've seen present well-grounded supporting research. Many of these authors slant their work toward men's core stability without considering sex-specific differences, and none consider the powerful influence of your mind and spirit on your health and resistance to injury. Unlike anything else yet published, this book provides an expert analysis of the current scientific understanding of holistic core health, because education is the key to injury prevention and lifelong wellness.

With this knowledge, you will have all the tools necessary to improve your core stability, health, and physical fitness, while significantly reducing your risk of injury. You'll also be able to teach what you know to other women and men who will benefit. You'll be able to actually prevent injuries and watch your physical performance in every area of life improve over time, instead of spending months or years working to recover from injuries and setbacks. Although you will never notice the ACL you didn't tear or the bone you didn't break, you will definitely notice your increased ability to perform in athletics and daily life because of your improved core stability. This paradigm shift in health, from treatment to prevention, will change the lives of millions of people for the better. I hope this book promotes widespread understanding of the power of a healthy core and its importance for a healthier, happier life for all human beings, from toddlers, to pro athletes, to the elderly.

Then, I'll teach you The Core BASE, an integrative, holistic guide for breathing, awareness, stability, and empowerment of your core in body, mind, and spirit. You will learn how to transform not just your body, but also your mindset and your life, through scientifically supported strategies. I'll show you the same evidence-based framework used in my research and practice so that you can clearly understand exactly what the science shows, and what you must do in order to reap the benefits of a healthy, stable core while reducing your risk of injuries. I'll do my best throughout this book to make the science as simple as possible so that you can truly master this information and apply it in your own life.

This is not just a 30-day workout plan or a short-term fix. You'll notice significant positive results from the Core BASE training within a few weeks, because that's what the research shows. And you'll continue to improve as you progress in your core training year after year, even if you're already an elite athlete.

Improve Your Health with an Integrative, Holistic Guide to Core Empowerment in Mind-Body-Spirit

"It takes more than a good-looking body. You've got to have the heart
and soul to go with it."
—Epictetus

Wouldn't you love to look and feel amazing—physically, emotionally, and spiritually—every single day? Do you dream about living without aches and pains? Do you hope to summon more strength for all of your current activities and sports? Would you like to try a new exercise class or sport without fear of injury? Do you want to take your triathlon or marathon performance to the next level? Can you imagine yourself with beautiful posture and grace through all of your movements? Are you on a never-ending mission to lose weight? Is the idea of having more energy and stamina enticing?

This book and training program will provide you with simple strategies to achieve all these benefits of a strong, stable, and resilient core. You'll discover science-based strategies and exercises for more effective breathing, mindful meditation, and dynamic stretching, plus fifty core strength and stability exercises, complementary strategies for core empowerment, and body awareness seeds of wisdom that you can easily integrate into your day to feel more strength, resilience, confidence, and energy.

Throughout my decades of clinical and investigative experience, I have learned that the foundation for injury prevention, recovery, and overall wellness is based on four fundamental principles of a healthy core BASE that each person must learn and incorporate into their life to truly flourish:

Breathing deeply with dynamic stretches to align and awaken your inner core. Without proper breathing habits, you will never maximize your core strength and stability.

Awareness of your mind-core connection through meditation, kinetic learning, and nervous system training with scientifically-based core exercises for activation, strength, coordination, and control.

Stability of your core as the control center of your body, developed through a dynamic core stability arsenal of exercises for your core to function properly and protect you from injury.

Empowerment of your core through alternative philosophies and activities that will help you make core stability part of your lifestyle. You'll be able to use your own unique interests and skills to achieve core empowerment while having fun and enjoying new adventures and challenges.

I am writing this book as a guide to help you explore and empower your core BASE so you can learn to live your life from your core, and harness and embrace your unlimited potential for strength, health, and growth.

Let's get started!

PART 1: CORE FUNDAMENTALS

CHAPTER 1

Understanding the Core

"All our knowledge begins with the senses,
proceeds then to understanding, and ends with reason."
—Immanuel Kant

Core stability is a very important concept, one I've spent my entire career studying—but if you only understand the concept intellectually, you won't really understand it completely. That's because you must combine the concept of core stability in your mind with your body's ability to perceive it. Without perception, you simply cannot achieve or maintain optimal core stability. This ability to perceive where each part of your body is and how it moves through space is called proprioception, and you're about to learn how to master it.

But first, let's make sure we are clear on the key concept of core stability, and that we aren't starting with some popular misconceptions. The concept of core stability has long been associated with health and wellness as an important component of living a long and healthy life. This buzzword has permeated health clubs, yoga studios, the internet, health and wellness publications, and scientific literature, but most of us still don't quite understand what core stability is or how to achieve it.

Defining Core Stability

> "At the center of your being you have the answer."
> —Lao Tzu

In the Western scientific world, the core has been described as the body's center of balance and strength. It includes thirty-five muscles (abdominal, back, pelvic, and glutes), plus the spine, pelvis, and hip joints. Eastern philosophies, from the Ancient Greeks to traditional Chinese and Indian yogi masters, have looked beyond the physical aspect of the core for thousands of years, attributing to it certain spiritual properties. These traditions claim that mastering the spiritual components of your core through practices like deep breathing, meditation, and moving your body into and out of different postures can help you achieve inner power and enlightenment. New scientific evidence supports the benefits of these Eastern complementary practices, such as meditation, yoga, and martial arts, and their abilities to improve your health and empower your core.

This new research, which we'll discuss in more detail later, has created a paradigm shift in modern integrated health because it has forced scientists and medical professionals to recognize the importance of the mind-body-spirit connection for optimal wellness and injury prevention. This new paradigm has created a symbiotic approach that draws from both Western (conventional) and Eastern (alternative and complementary) philosophies to understand a person's unique set of circumstances and address their full range of physical, psychological, social, environmental, and spiritual influences. Science has shown us that merging some of the best practices from Western and Eastern healing modalities is the best way to improve core stability and overall health.

Until recently, if an athlete tore a muscle in their shoulder while pitching a baseball, surgery would repair the tear, and the rehabilitation would focus on strengthening the repaired muscle. Now, we are finally recognizing the importance of prevention, because most of these types of injuries can be prevented. Science has also shown that we must focus not only on rehabilitating the injury itself, but training and educating the athlete in many areas, including their body awareness, biomechanics, psychological motivators, and lifestyle choices such as self-care, nutrition, and sleep. We must take a holistic approach to physical training, injury prevention, and injury rehabilitation in order to get the best results.

The formal laboratory definition of core stability that I developed in my groundbreaking medical research is "the foundation of dynamic trunk control that allows production, transfer, and control of force and motion to distal segments of the body." In simpler terms, core stability is the ability to set your body into motion and control your body throughout this motion by using your core muscles to move the way you intend to, whether you're hitting a perfect tennis forehand shot, running a marathon, or playing with your children.

Core stability is also the ability to control your muscles unconsciously in order to stabilize yourself, like if you trip on a rock or the root of a tree while hiking in the forest. Without core stability, you will not be able to do the things you want to do with your body nearly as effectively or safely, and when you do trip or lose your balance, you are much more likely to get injured.

You actually can't make any significant movements without using your core muscles and joints. It is the activation of your core muscles that propels your body through space, whether you're walking your dog, picking a pen up off the floor, or playing sports. Want to twist off the lid from that jar of pickles? You may think all you have to do is twist it with your arms, but you need core muscle activation to do that. No core muscle activation means no opening jars for you.

Scientists have been studying how the body moves and functions for years, and what we've found is that this sequence of trunk (torso) muscle activation prior to muscle activation in the arms and legs is evident in all daily movements, beginning from the time you're born until the day you die. Want to jump higher, throw a ball faster, or run farther? You need your core muscles to be in tip-top shape to do that. Contracting the core muscles in just the right way at just the right time provides the stable foundation for moving your body the way you intend to.

But sometimes, your body will have to move in ways you don't consciously intend to, like when you're walking and don't see a crack in the sidewalk, so your ankle twists in an awkward way. These are the moments when injuries can either occur or be prevented, and that all depends on your body's capacity to maintain or resume the correct position of your trunk following perturbation. Perturbation, or a challenge to the core, could be a bumpy car ride, a pull from a dog's leash, an unexpected shove at a crowded concert, or a sudden change in direction to avoid an oncoming soccer opponent. If your body isn't prepared or able to properly readjust its positioning after perturbation, you could lose your balance, take a hard fall, or suffer a serious injury. You certainly won't be able to perform at your best if that happens.

Your Core Hardware

"It's not the beauty of the building you should look at; it is the construction of the foundation that will stand the test of time."
—David Allen Coe

Most people think of the core as the sculpted six-pack abs seen in ads, but it actually includes all the muscles of your trunk, pelvis, and hips. This includes the abdominal muscles (the six-pack), back extensors (which run along your spine), obliques (which wrap diagonally around your waist), transversus abdominis (the broad muscle around your trunk that allows you to suck in your stomach), multifidi (which connect the vertebrae, or segments of your spine, to each other), quadratus lumborum (which connects your ribs, spine and pelvis), diaphragm (the breathing muscle below your lungs), the muscles of your pelvic floor, and your hip muscles.

"Think global, act local" is a motto often used in environmental conservation efforts. To consider our impact on the entire planet's health, we are asked to act locally in our own communities and cities. This concept also relates to the health of your core, as core muscles are classified as "global" and "local." Global muscles and local muscles behave differently from each other and fulfill completely different roles in your body. Local core muscles are deep and closest to the bones, while the global muscles are more superficial. The global muscles make up the shapely form you see in athletes and sports enthusiasts.

When you see a buff Olympic swimmer making large, strong strokes in the water, you can see the definition of their hard-working global muscles, including the abs (your trunk flexors), lats (the largest muscles of your upper body that connect your torso and arms), erector spinae (the spine extensors that run parallel to the spine), and glutes (the most powerful muscle group in your body). These large, outer muscles connect the pelvis, ribs, and limbs; produce high forces and large movements; and indirectly affect the vertebrae (the bones in your spine), supporting them as the prime movers.

What you don't see are the inner muscles such as the diaphragm, pelvic floor, transversus abdominis, and multifidus, which are the deeper stabilizing muscles that control individual vertebral segments with precision. These inner muscles produce lower forces over longer periods of time, supporting posture by stabilizing the segments of your spine and providing involuntary, automatic adjustments in posture prior to movement. In normal function, these deep muscles have the ability to automatically and simultaneously activate before and during any movement to control the center of your body. This important inner core squad of muscles prepares you for movement by anticipating impending forces to your trunk.

In order to do this, these local muscles need to have sufficient activation and strength to create stiffness in the spine before you move your trunk, arms, or legs, like the tensioned cable wires of a ship or free-standing tower (Figure 1). Each muscle that surrounds the spine must provide a certain amount of tension to maintain the stability of the spine, prevent buckling and injury, and provide efficient, effective, and powerful movement.

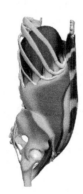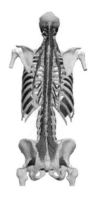

Figure 1. Key muscles of the inner core hardware from the side and back views. Source: Medical Historical Library, Harvey Cushing/ John Hay Whitney Medical Library, Yale University.

While the global core muscles of a sculpted physique get all the glory, the local muscles quietly work behind the scenes to anticipate your next move and activate appropriately to support you, fine-tune your movement, and save you from injury. It is through the balance and synergistic cooperation of both the global and the local muscles that true core stability, with intersegmental control of your spine, is achieved. This is what the Core BASE Guide will teach you. Instead of simply focusing on building a better six-pack, you'll discover the keys to building a foundation of core strength, stability, and coordination that will allow you to perform better in extreme sports and in everyday activities (and build a six-pack too, if that's what you're looking for).

Finding Your Core Hardware

"Hardware will give you the power."
—Akshat Paul

The first step to achieving a strong, functional core is to connect with each of your core muscles by learning to find them and feel them as they work, since you cannot strengthen a muscle that your brain is not using. Let's try some simple techniques to acquaint you with the key muscles of your core hardware that you probably don't consciously contract. Most people are familiar with the big, global muscles, so let's first introduce you to those outer muscles.

Sit comfortably with your shoulders, head, and neck relaxed. Place your hands on your belly while you slightly flex or curl forward, feeling the tightness in your abs. Next, place your hands on your back with your fingers on the muscles that run along each side of your spine, the erector spinae. Feel these long back extensors (your "I Love Standing" muscles: iliocostalis, longissimus, and spinalis) as you arch backwards or even push your shoulders into the back of a chair to really get these large muscles to pop out. In addition to extending your spine, these powerful muscles side-bend and stabilize your spine and your pelvis. To feel your obliques, cross your arms and spread your fingers just below your ribcage while you side-bend and twist your trunk from side to side. Say hello to your glutes by squeezing your cheeks together.

Your quadratus lumborum muscles, the deepest abdominal muscles of the back, span from the back of your pelvis to your lower ribs, connecting your ribcage, the top of your pelvis, and the bones of your spine. This pair of important muscles stabilizes the ribs, improves efficiency of the diaphragm, and extends your spine when working in unison. Independently, each of these muscles function to side-bend your trunk and to move and control your pelvis. Find one of your quadratus lumborum muscles by standing up tall and placing your hands on your hips. Place your thumbs on your back, halfway between your waist and your spine, pressing in the space between your bottom rib and your hip. You can feel the muscle engage as you hike the same-side hip by slightly lifting the same-side leg a couple inches off the ground.

Your quadratus lumborum muscles also work together with your psoas muscles—the long, thick muscles deep in your abdomen that connect the front of your spine to your thighs—to stabilize, decompress, and support your spine, especially when bearing heavy loads, like when you lift or jump. Your psoas muscles are deep in your torso, three to four inches beneath your skin. To find them, place your hands on your abdomen at the level of your hip bones and work slightly away from your navel to your sides. You can sense these deep pulleys activating when you initiate the movement of lifting your knee toward your chest.

In this book you'll learn how to strengthen and coordinate not just these large global muscles, but also your inner core, local muscles so you can achieve maximum stability and prevent injuries. Learning to activate your inner core begins with your breath. To get a feel for these important muscles, place one hand on your upper chest and the other right below your rib cage. Breathe in slowly and deeply through your nose so that your belly moves out against your hand to activate your diaphragm, the muscle at the base of your lungs and the roof of your core.

To promote a stronger contraction of your diaphragm, try applying some gentle pressure with your lower hand to resist your inhalation. You may also try breathing out through pursed lips, like you are blowing up a balloon or blowing through a straw, for more diaphragmatic activation on exhalation. The diaphragm plays a critical role in all of your body's functioning by leading the charge to get the inner core squad firing.

Notice how when you take a deep breath in, your ribcage opens to the front, sides, and back, and your abdomen expands. This expansion turns on your transversus abdominis, the deepest of your abdominal muscles, which runs horizontally and wraps all the way around your abdomen circumferentially under your obliques. You can activate your transverse abdominis muscles by drawing your belly button toward your spine as you exhale the deep breath out, imagining the broad, sheet-like muscles tightening around your core to force all the air out. Place your hands on your hips with your fingertips on the pointy protrusions of your pelvis and slide them slightly inward and downward. Here you can feel for firmness as your transversus abdominis activates from deep within your abdomen.

Activation of your transversus abdominis muscles is automatically, synergistically coupled with the rise of your pelvic floor (which can be felt with contractions, like when you stop your flow of pee), and the small, but very important spinal multifidus muscles. The multifidus muscles are a bit trickier to feel, as they lie deep in between the bones of your spine. These little guys play an important role in stabilizing your core from behind the scenes of your outer back muscles.

Get to know your multifidus muscles by lying on your stomach with a pillow under your belly. You can best feel them deep along the sides of your spine in your lower back, as you begin lifting your arms or legs slightly off the ground. These deep muscles also fire when you think about drawing the dimples of your lower back together and initiate the movement of arching your back without actually arching it. If you do arch your back, this will engage the large, global, superficial back extensors too much to allow you to feel the subtle bulge of the deep multifidus muscles. To ramp up the firing of the multifidus, activate your pelvic floor and transversus abdominis while taking an even deeper breath, and fully engage your inner core squad of muscles that are working in unison.

Developing awareness of these inner core muscles may be a challenge at first, but learning to feel, activate, and understand the action of these individual muscles is an important first step in training the neural pathways of your whole core team of muscles. These neural pathways are critical for coordinated action so all the core muscles can work in harmony. They lengthen, brace, and maintain the shape of your spine so your "core can do your chores." Don't worry if you can't feel some of these muscles activating right now; it can take time to gain this kind of proprioceptive awareness, and you will continue to improve as you practice more and implement the Core BASE training program.

Your Core Software

"Software is the magic thing whose importance only goes up over time."
—Bill Gates

If you think of your body's core team of muscles as your hardware, then your nervous system is your core software. You can only achieve optimal core health if your software is programmed to turn on all of your local and global core muscles in the right way at the right time. The timing of all these muscle contractions is critical because strength alone is not sufficient for core stability when you're moving around in the real world. Strength is the ability to produce and maintain force throughout a movement; stability, on the other hand, is the ability to resist unwanted movement, which requires a far more complex set of software instructions than simply doing a sit-up or bench press.

So, if you have strength in your trunk muscles, you may be able to do a lot of sit-ups or back extensions, but when you need to stabilize your core to meet real functional demands (like carrying a heavy bag of groceries), you need neuromuscular control to stabilize your spine, maintain optimal alignment between your spine and other body parts, and prevent unwanted, potentially dangerous movements that can set you up for injury. Strength without proper neuromuscular control will not protect you from injuries and might even make you more likely to suffer one.

Neuromuscular control is the ability to coherently engage all of your trunk muscles in harmony so you can achieve core stability, and it's specific to the task being performed. Even a very small alteration in the angle, speed, or direction of your movement may create a significant change in the way your core muscles must activate to protect your body from an injury. The contribution and timing of each trunk muscle's contractions continually change through every movement you make to achieve the necessary balance between stability and mobility for all your body parts. Together, the core muscles create a natural back brace before and during movement to support your spine as you bend, twist, lift, and move through life with optimal performance and avoidance of injury. An injury to your spinal cord could be life threatening, so your core muscles have evolved to do everything possible to prevent such an injury.

Over time, the core muscles can become weakened and less able to do their job for a number of reasons, including inactivity, poor posture, or injury. This leads to dysfunctional movement patterns, which further increase the risk of pain and injury. Core muscle actions must be precisely timed and coordinated to occur at the right moment, for the correct duration, and with the right combination of forces to stabilize your spine.

The most recent discoveries demonstrate that proper core training facilitates software and hardware adaptations that provide stabilization through muscular pre-activation and reactive patterns that protect your body from injurious forces. This requires neuromuscular strategies that you will develop with the Core BASE Guide to control, direct, and maximize all of your movements for efficiency, effectiveness, and safety, whether you're playing with your kids or competing in the NBA finals.

How to Keep Your Core Stable

"When you can't control what's happening, challenge yourself to
control the way you respond to what's happening.
That's where your true power is."
—Karen Salmansohn

To achieve core stability, there are three primary neuromuscular requirements that must be met. First, your core position must be internally observable, meaning you must be able to sense the position of your body both consciously and unconsciously. In order for you to actually know where your body is in space, your core must provide your brain (the control center) with accurate information about the position of your body. This information is obtained from sensors in your joints and muscles, and influenced by quick reflexive reactions (that you don't control), as well as voluntary reactions (that you do control).

Second, this information must be accurately relayed to and from the brain through your nerves. This information is then used by the brain to generate appropriate control to the core muscles to make the proper adjustments so you can move your body the way you need to without getting injured. Your nervous system is the messenger service between awareness and control of your muscles.

Third, the system must be controlled. Your core is controlled by feed-forward and feedback mechanisms. Feed-forward refers to proactive, preparatory neuromuscular strategies that your central nervous system computes for the right preparatory core muscle activation in all your movements. For example, when I walk outside in the slippery New England snow, I subconsciously adjust my usual walking pattern to take shorter, more careful steps with this anticipatory strategy.

Feedback control is reactive to core awareness relative to your surroundings. This comes into play when you hit a super slippery patch of ice, or when any other kind of disturbance to your original projected motion sends sensory information to recalculate muscle activation. Your core muscles must have enough power to provide quick and accurate corrections in all directions to help you regain your balance in your posture or trajectory of movement.

Problems in any of these areas can lead to core instability, resulting in uncontrollable motions of your body. This means that the body may be unexpectedly displaced beyond its safe physiologic limits, causing physical damage or injury to your muscles, joints, or soft tissues. All three are important components of a stable core, and they'll be developed with the training of the Core BASE Guide.

Think of a marionette with moveable parts on strings, that moves by the grace of a puppet master. The puppet master is the brain that controls the body segments to orchestrate specific movements in the puppet. The strings are like your nerves that must work together to control opposable forces and operate each segment, and the segments must all work together to achieve the desired movement. When the puppet master moves one string, several joints move at once, which is the same way your body works, because it's all connected. As John Muir so aptly observed, "When one tugs at a single thing in nature, one finds it attaches to the rest of the world."

Like a marionette, the body is a multi-segmental system. Each joint in your body, from your head to your toes, is one segment in this system. Forces and motions generated at one joint affect all of the remaining joints. Thus, problems in the control or stability of one segment may harm the performance of the other segments, to the point that your body may become unstable and susceptible to injury. Because your core muscles are the ones that must activate first in order to initiate any major movement of your body, any loss of stability in your core may cause instability in every area of your body from your head to your feet.

My published biomechanical research on hundreds of Yale University collegiate athletes has determined that poor core stability increases the risk of injury. This is the science of biomechanics: it doesn't matter if you're running, throwing, or dunking a basketball; your core muscles must activate first in order for you to move the way you want for optimal performance with reduced risk of injury.

The significant core stability predictors of injury, or the measurable reasons for getting injured, are impaired core proprioception (awareness) and core control (response), which I will now explain to you.

Defining Proprioception

"All our knowledge begins with our senses."
—Immanuel Kant

Proprioception, sometimes known as your "sixth sense," is the ability to sense the location and movement of your body. It's what allows your core to be internally observable. The cumulative sensory input of proprioception to your brain is the reason you are able to move without consciously thinking about your surroundings. This ability plays an important role in every move you make, as it's this awareness that allows you to touch your nose, balance on one leg, walk through your house in the dark, put your hair up with your eyes closed, or catch a football.

I witnessed one of the most amazing examples of proprioceptive ability as a student intern for a nursing home rehabilitation center. One of the physical therapists working there was blind. She had not only completed her degree and license with this disability, but was successfully treating patients who had strokes, amputations, and brain injuries. She was teaching them how to move and walk again, so not only did she have to worry about her own balance, but another person's balance and stability were literally in her hands. Proprioception is actually enhanced in the visually impaired, as they learn to adapt and navigate the world without sight. But you don't have to go blind to improve your proprioception: you'll be able to do that using the exercises in this book.

When you move, your brain senses the position, effort, and force of your actions and movements, then directs your body to respond accordingly with core control. To clarify these concepts even more, I will describe the methods that I used in my studies to quantify core awareness and core control, and describe how you can simulate our laboratory testing to assess your own ability for these two critical factors.

Core Awareness Lab Testing

We measured core awareness using a seated apparatus, which passively rotated our subjects away from the starting position at a slow, steady speed, then briefly held the subject in that position.

Proprioception was tested when we disengaged the motor, allowing the subject to rotate back. The subject stopped the apparatus by pressing a switch when they felt like they were back in the starting position. Some subjects were able to accurately perceive where their body was in space, while others who thought they were back in a neutral position were actually still twisted and out of alignment. When these athletes were monitored throughout their years at Yale, deficits in core awareness were observed in those who sustained injuries and compared with uninjured athletes from the same varsity sports teams.

Core Awareness Self-Assessment

It's time to try a quick exercise that will help you assess your own proprioceptive abilities. Sit or stand in front of a mirror and observe the position of your trunk. Fold your arms across your chest, close your eyes, and slowly twist only your upper body in one direction, turning your shoulders as far as you can without allowing your hips to shift. Pause briefly in this position (two to three seconds). Then, while keeping your eyes closed, slowly rotate your upper body back until you feel like your body has returned to your starting position. Open your eyes and observe the actual position of your trunk, then mentally compare this to your original position. Repeat the same task on the opposite side, noting any differences in your accuracy from one side to the other. This demonstrates your trunk's inherent awareness, or proprioception, which works in tandem with core control, or response, to achieve stability.

Core Control

"To expect the unexpected shows a thoroughly modern intellect."
—Oscar Wilde

Having a hard time lugging your groceries up the stairs? Feeling a bit wobbly when you walk on a rocky beach? Is your yoga tree pose swaying in the wind? Core control is the essence of every move you make, and it's critical for maintaining your balance in all activities. Your body has three feedback systems that provide information to your brain to help you keep your balance. The first is the vestibular system located in your inner ear, which acts like a carpenter's level for your body. The second component of balance is proprioception from your muscles and joints, which provides awareness of your core. The third coordinator of balance is your vision, which also sends information to your brain about your body's position.

Your brain assimilates all of this information to activate your trunk muscles for the necessary adjustments to maintain your balance, and this process creates the phenomenon that we call core control. Daily activities and sports are unpredictable: ice on the driveway, a discarded banana peel, or an unexpected shove can surprise you without any warning. Because you don't always know when you will need to react, you need to be prepared so you can react efficiently. Core control before, during, and after an unexpected perturbation is necessary to protect you from any unforeseen safety hazards, collisions, or extreme adjustments in movement from sudden disturbances. You can significantly improve your core control by increasing your proprioception and upgrading your software with proper core training.

Core Control Lab Testing

In our studies, we also tested the same collegiate athletes for core control by measuring trunk displacement (or how far the subject's trunk moved before the subject stopped and corrected the motion) using a sudden force release apparatus. In this core control testing apparatus, the subjects sat in a chair that was able to tip over in different directions (front to back, and side to side). A cable, attached to a chest harness and held in place with an electromagnet, served as a resisting force to stabilize the subject. The cable was then released at random time intervals. Deficits in core control, measured by trunk displacements, were greater in athletes who later sustained injury. These findings establish the link between poor core stability and injury, and provide valuable insight into the role of core awareness and core control for health and wellness.

Core Control Self-Assessment

To better understand the concept of core control, try sitting on top of a pile of pillows or cushions. To add perturbation (or a challenge to your position), try balancing a book on top of your head, or throw a ball up in the air or against a wall and catch it. This assessment will help you see how well you can control and stabilize your core.

I asked all of my graduate research students to practice this in our classroom. They sat on a stable surface with their legs dangling, noticing how stable they felt in this position. The students practiced tossing balls to each other and giving each other friendly shoves. Next, I had them do the same exercise on an unstable surface. Since we had a room full of Physical Therapy equipment, the students experimented with large exercise balls, wobble boards, and cushions, and noted the variability in their core control with different surfaces, different sizes and weights of balls, and different velocities and angles of throwing and catching, which all imposed variable forces on the trunk and required unique core activation strategies.

Don't be discouraged or disappointed if you find from these self-assessments that you don't have great control of your core. I will teach you the skills you need to face the perturbations of everyday life. Core awareness and core control are interdependent and must work together for each and every movement you make. In order to prevent serious injuries, you must be able to maintain your core position or trajectory as you move, change direction, or make any kind of quick movements. The ability to control your body in this way is critically important, whether you're catching some air on your mountain bike or catching yourself when your foot slides on a slippery floor.

In the next chapter, you'll learn about the biomechanics of the core so you can understand how to move your body in ways that are more effective, which will help you reduce your risk of injuries and pain.

Seeds for Thought

- Were you able to identify your core muscles and feel them contracting and relaxing? Did you discover new muscles you weren't aware of before?

- Are you aware of the position of your trunk throughout the day?

- How can you incorporate deep breathing, meditation, and movement into your daily life?

- Have you ever suffered an injury because you unexpectedly lost your balance or stability?

- How do you think your overall performance in sports and daily activities could be improved with better core awareness and control?

CHAPTER 2

Core Biomechanics

"A chain is only as strong as its weakest link."
—English proverb

Balancing Sticks to Understand Core Stability

A team is only as strong as its weakest player, and core control is the MVP of your body's team. The structure, function, and motion of your core's mechanical aspects can be easily understood with a simple activity. In this exercise, you'll be balancing a stick in the palm of your hand. You can try this exercise using a broom handle, mop, chopstick, or a straight stick from your backyard. Your goal is simple: balance the stick in the palm of your hand.

When the stick's center of mass is directly under the base (your palm), the system is balanced in a state of equilibrium and no corrective forces are required. When the stick starts to fall, your hand must move to catch it. The necessary size and speed of the hand movements are related to the size and speed of stick displacement, with larger and faster stick displacement requiring larger and faster hand movements to bring it back into balance.

In order to make those larger and faster hand movements required to balance the stick, you must apply greater forces to your hand by contracting your muscles even more. If you were trying to balance the stick with your eyes closed, this task would be much more difficult because vision provides additional feedback about the position of the stick so that you can respond more quickly as it begins to fall in any given direction. With a faster counter-balancing response, less displacement occurs, and less force is required to maintain stability.

That's why core control and proprioception are so important: the better your proprioception and core control, the less work your body has to do in order to maintain balance and accomplish everyday tasks. That means your muscles, bones, tendons, and ligaments will not have to endure the extreme forces that someone with less proprioception and core control would have to endure.

For an extra challenge, you can try the stick-balancing exercise after adding a small weight on the top of the stick to increase the destabilizing mass. By adding more weight to the top of the stick, you've raised its center of gravity and made the task of balancing it much more difficult, requiring more speed and larger movements of your hand in order to keep it balanced.

These simple exercises clearly demonstrate the point that greater forces acting on the stick are necessary to maintain stability when the quality of awareness or control is weakened, or when you raise the center of gravity. Your body is just like that stick. In order to avoid falling over, your core must make constant adjustments in order to maintain your balance. If that didn't happen, you would just fall over instead of being able to stand up!

Under static conditions, such as standing, small control impairments may not result in any significant forces or displacements. Under dynamic conditions such as jumping, landing, and cutting, which magnify destabilizing forces acting on your body, these forces and displacements significantly increase, compromising your control and leaving you more susceptible to injury.

Notice how there are several important factors involved here that determine your core control. First is proprioception: the more awareness you have of your body's position in space, the faster and more accurately you'll be able to respond when your body is out of balance, thus reducing the forces required to stabilize yourself. Next is the center of gravity: the higher your center of gravity is, the more likely you are to lose your balance, or need to make larger and more forceful movements to regain your balance. And finally, core control: the more forcefully and effectively your body is able to move in response to a perturbation or loss of balance, the easier it will be for your body to maintain its balance.

The Core is the Central Link of the Kinetic Chain

"You have been told that even like a chain, you are as weak as your weakest link. This is but half the truth. You are also as strong as the strongest link."
—Kahlil Gibran

It's important to understand what your body's kinetic chain is, and how the core is the central link of this chain. Your body is an amazing machine comprised of over 650 muscles, all working together to get you out of bed, through your daily tasks, and across the finish line. Your trunk, or core, is the most important link that connects the upper links (shoulders, elbows, wrists, and fingers) with your lower links (hips, knees, ankles, and toes). The entire kinetic chain is the system by which all of your muscles work together in your body to function efficiently.

As an anatomy student and teacher, I have spent much time learning and teaching the movements of each of these muscles. For instance, the function of your rectus abdominis (your abs) is to flex or bend your trunk, as when you do a crunch, with the muscle shortening as the two connection points come closer together (a concentric contraction).

Yet, the same muscle must also provide stability as it lengthens (eccentric contraction) and the two connection points of the muscle move further apart. During this lengthening contraction, your abs work as a braking mechanism, slowing down and controlling your motion, like when you jump or catch yourself from falling.

This same muscle also works isometrically throughout your day with constant tension when you maintain a static position, meaning the muscle length does not change (like when you sit, do a plank, or try to hold on to a ball against the pressure of an opponent trying to strip it away).

In reality, core stability in daily life is dependent upon all three of these types of contractions (concentric, eccentric, and isometric) working in concert with the rest of the body. Think of how your abs feel after riding on a motorcycle, waterskiing, raking, or laughing too hard. The function of your abdominals, in addition to bending your trunk, is also to provide a foundation of stability for all movement by contracting at just the right time, in just the right way, with just the right amount of tension.

Isolated exercises like crunches or sit-ups may help you get well-defined abs, but they can actually cause imbalances in your kinetic chain and leave you more vulnerable to injuries over time. Doing these exercises alone will not train all of your core muscles on the front, side, and back of your body to balance and work in coordination with your body's chain like they do in real situations.

Think about it: how often in life do you need to bend over with the same significant speed or force of contracting your abs as you do when performing crunches? Not very often. But you will need your abs to stabilize your body countless times throughout every day of your life as you move. Rather than working on outdated exercise programs without scientific backing, you will learn to fire all of your core muscles that take your body's chain through all planes of motion (up, down, left, right, front, and back), with your core muscles controlling multiple joints at the same time and working together in perfect orchestration. You will also learn exercises that will ensure your muscles get better at concentric, eccentric, and isometric contractions. Developing your core as the central link of your kinetic chain will allow you to develop a much better level of fitness for everything you want to do in life.

The Importance of a Balanced Chain

"Balance of the body is the foundation for balance in life."
—B.K.S. Iyengar

Your posterior chain refers to the muscles located on the back side of your body, including the muscles of your back, glutes, and hamstrings. Prolonged sitting, sleeping in a fetal position, and many forms of exercise (even walking and running) disproportionately shorten the anterior, or front muscles, of the body. Our modern lifestyles often force us into a position where our necks are craned forward, our shoulders are shrugged up toward our ears, our backs are rounded, and our hands are out in front of us. Over time, this tightens the muscles on the front of your body and weakens the muscles on the back of your body. Weakening of these muscles makes it difficult for them to activate properly, which predisposes us to imbalance, poor posture, and injury.

Even bodybuilders and athletes often suffer from a neglected posterior chain, also known as "dormant bottom syndrome" or "gluteal amnesia." Your "mirror muscles" are all located on the front of your body, so you probably tend to give them more attention, neglecting the muscles on the back of your body. In fact, most people simply don't address the posterior chain when exercising because they focus their training on "beach muscles" (biceps, pecs, and abs), but neglect to train the body parts that truly develop balanced strength and stability.

For many years people relied on sit-ups as the main exercise for their cores, but sit-ups and crunches exert massive compressive forces on the spinal discs and contribute to pain and injury. They're not very natural movements for human beings. Overemphasis on the "mirror muscles" causes anterior dominance and posterior dormancy, meaning the muscles on the front of the body are more awake and developed than the sleepy ones on the back. It's important to emphasize well-rounded training for optimal human functioning and core health.

Your glutes play a vital role in how your body functions, as they are the biggest, most powerful muscle group in your body and are key to maintaining alignment, stability, support, and shock absorption of your entire body's chain. When your posterior muscles fail to absorb shock during activities, this results in overloading the rest of your joints. Weak glutes are a common issue and often a root cause of injuries throughout the entire body. They can cause pain in your feet, legs, knees, back, or elsewhere.

Signs of a Sleepy Posterior Chain

"Chains of habit are generally too small to be felt until they are too strong to be broken."
—Samuel Johnson

Look at your standing posture in the mirror from the side and back, or snap a selfie in the mirror. Are you slouched forward? Do you have a "pancake butt?" Do you have stocky quads on the front of your thighs, but not well-defined hamstrings on the back of your thighs? When you lie flat on your back, do the muscles on the front of your body feel tight? Are your shoulders slightly raised off the ground? When you bring one knee towards your chest, does your other leg lift off the ground? These are all signs of an anterior/posterior chain imbalance. A tight anterior chain, combined with a stretched or sleepy posterior chain, will not give you the balance and stability you need for optimal functioning of your body.

Another way to check how well the important muscles of your posterior chain are performing is to stand in front of a mirror on one foot and lift the other leg off the ground. If your posterior chain kicks in like it is supposed to, your pelvis will remain level. However, if your posterior chain is not living up to its potential, your pelvis will drop down on the side of your leg that's in the air. Lifting your right leg tests your left posterior chain, and lifting the left leg tests the right posterior chain.

By strengthening your posterior chain, you can improve your slouch, reduce your risk of developing pain, and boost your sense of physical confidence. When there is an imbalance between the anterior and posterior chains, you are more likely to sustain injuries such as rotator cuff tears, hamstring strains, knee ligament injuries, and back pain. Luckily a dormant posterior chain is not a life sentence! The Core BASE Guide will reboot your glutes, improve your posture and balance, and prevent injury in all aspects of your life, including sports. Don't worry if the posterior aspect of your core has been asleep—I'll teach you how to wake it up!

Neuromuscular Imbalances

"The desire for symmetry, for balance, for rhythm . . . is one of the most inveterate of human instincts."
–Edith Wharton

As a physical therapist, one of the hardest things to explain to a patient is that their knee, foot, shoulder, or elbow pain is actually being caused by issues with their core muscle function. Most people are not aware of their own trunk deficits or imbalances—not even avid fitness enthusiasts and high-level athletes! In fact, in my experience, the most elite athletes tend to have huge imbalances throughout their bodies that can predispose them to serious injuries. This is especially common in quarterbacks, pitchers, tennis players, basketball players who favor a specific sided lay-up, and soccer players who prefer to kick with one leg. Most athletes have a preferred plant leg, a preferred drive leg when propelling the body into a single leg jump, or a preferred leg to land on. These side-to-side differences tend to be greater in injured athletes, and are even more exaggerated in injured women compared to injured men.

Almost all of us have a dominant arm and leg, as well as preferred movement patterns that can create imbalances throughout our body's kinetic chain and predispose us to injuries. For example, you may prefer to write with your right hand, or kick with your left leg. Only 1 percent of us are ambidextrous, or equally capable and skillful with both sides of the body. Some famous ambidextrous people include Leonardo Da Vinci, Benjamin Franklin, and Albert Einstein—but you don't need to be a brilliant artist, a famous statesman, or a genius to train yourself to use both arms and legs with equal skill. A house painter once surprised me with his efficiency using a brush in each hand!

Everyone knows their dominant arm, but your dominant leg may not be so obvious, unless you're a soccer player. To find your dominant leg, put your "best foot forward." Have someone give you a friendly shove from behind, and your dominant leg will be the one you step forward with. This leg is usually bigger and stronger, and used more for finer motor skills, whereas your non-dominant leg is usually better at balancing your center of mass, like when you prepare to kick, jump, or swing a golf club.

Neuromuscular imbalances may also be related to an old injury or lack of muscle flexibility (limberness), timing (anticipatory muscle activity), activation (ability to turn on), strength (ability to generate force), power (force production over a short period of time) and/or endurance (ability to sustain force). All of these factors can compromise your control over your body.

Your core muscles are activated by reflexes that respond to your actions and reactions. While many of your arm and leg movements are planned out, the movements of your core are reflex-driven, and they attempt to stabilize your trunk to protect you from injury and produce more efficient movement patterns. Imbalances in your body force your core to compensate. When the core has to compensate, your reflex reactions are interrupted and become less efficient and effective, leaving you more susceptible to injury.

Assess Your Entire Kinetic Chain

Right now, take a ten-minute break from reading to assess yourself for any imbalances in your body, from your toes to your neck. Head to a private room, take your clothes off, and observe your motion in front of the mirror while you do a closed chain activity, such as sitting down in a chair, squatting, or stepping down from a stool. Look for any noticeable side-to-side differences: Are your kneecaps "kissing each other" by collapsing into a knock-kneed position? Do you put more weight on one leg than the other? Does your trunk lean or rotate on the way up or down? These are all signs of imbalances that may throw your chain out of balance and predispose you to injuries.

Imbalances can occur in your upper body as well. Try raising your arms overhead like a snow-angel. Does one shoulder shrug up higher than the other? Imagine your arm as a crane and your trunk as the base of the crane. Just as the crane requires a stable base for it to function properly, it's important that your core is strong and stable so it can help anchor the arm for it to work efficiently, and for you to lift your arm up fully with good mechanics. If you have issues in your core, the muscles on top of your shoulder tend to overwork to compensate, causing mechanical imbalance, fatigue, and potential injury.

Ideally, the left and right sides of your body should be in the same plane relative to the ground. For example, your right hip shouldn't be any higher than your left hip. A push-up is another simple way to detect asymmetries of your trunk musculature in the mirror. If traditional push-ups are too difficult for you, try a modified version on your knees, or push against a high counter. Signs of core imbalances include a dipping down of your low back, or rotation of your body to one side or the other. The push-up should be executed in one fluid movement with a balanced and stable core.

Next, sit up in a chair and notice if your weight is evenly distributed on both legs, or if you shift your weight to one side. You can also try kneeling on one leg, then switching onto the other leg. Is it easier on one side than the other? Do you feel less secure or less balanced on one side? Don't be alarmed if you do detect imbalances; I'll show you how to correct them properly in the next section, and in the Core BASE Guide. You can also find more resources and video demonstrations at www.doczaz.com.

Correcting Imbalances

"When you pay attention, everything is your teacher."
–Ezra Bayda

To balance out these side-to-side differences, start by paying closer attention to how you move throughout your daily life. Do you always open a door with the same hand, or reach up to a high shelf with the same arm?

Try switching the roles of your dominant and non-dominant body parts by using your phone or opening a jar with your non-preferred hand, or switching to your non-preferred leg for your first step up a flight of stairs. If you like to ride, try switching between your "goofy" foot (left forward) and "regular" foot (right forward) on a snowboard, skateboard, or surfboard. Make an effort to consciously use your non-preferred side more often to avoid significant imbalances in your muscles, nerves, ligaments, and bones that develop over time. You'll be surprised to see how much you can train ambidexterity into your neuromuscular system!

Self-observation and awareness are critical for identifying the imbalances and deficits throughout every part of your body. The exercises I will teach you in this book will correct any imbalances you may have to get your body's chain in gear. Although it may seem counterintuitive, the more single-sided activities you perform (on both sides), the more side-to-side symmetry is restored. The human body possesses complex neurologic mechanisms to achieve balance, with maximal cross-over effects achieved when both sides of your body are alternately trained in single-limb activities. Additionally, single-limb activities influence synergistic recruitment of the posterior chain musculature to balance out asymmetries and decrease your risk of injury throughout your kinetic chain.

Get Your Core in Sync with Your Kinetic Chain

"Until you make the unconscious conscious, it will direct your life
and you will call it fate."
—Carl Jung

Think of your body's kinetic chain and how it functions when you perform a simple task, such as walking. When you step forward with your left foot, your right arm simultaneously swings forward. Following your left foot, your left knee moves forward, which also brings your left hip forward, causing your pelvis to rotate to the right, so your left hip is now in front of the right, and your trunk rotates to the right. Think of what happens when you wring out a towel: when you twist the top to the right and the bottom to the left, this creates torsion in the middle.

When your trunk twists while walking or running, your core muscles shorten, lengthen, and fire in synchrony with your upper and lower limbs. For something as simple as walking, core stability is required to achieve balance with the movement of each step forward. Imagine what your core does with five thousand steps each day, or with running, swimming, or other complex movements. Each of those muscles in your core is contracting thousands or even tens of thousands of times every single day. And if they're not able to function optimally, you won't be able to function optimally, either.

The Core BASE exercises will develop your strength and endurance to allow you to maintain good postural positions, and to execute even the most complex movement patterns with your core working in sync with your entire body. Your brain must train and coordinate each of your trunk muscles to create purposeful, efficient, precise activation so you can move your body the way you want without getting hurt. Establishing this harmony between your core muscles will improve the performance of all segments of your kinetic chain to create a symphony of safe and powerful movements. Every move you make in your daily life will be easier and safer when you train your core to do its job well.

Because every part of your body is connected from top to bottom, movement in any part of your body will create displacements or movements throughout the rest of it. This means that if you do not have good core control, other segments of your body must compensate by exerting larger forces and undergoing larger displacements or movements to maintain stability—and these greater forces and displacements transmitted through the entire body are what make the system susceptible to injury. Injury will occur at the weakest link, where the joint position is compromised, or the forces are close to tissue failure (like the knee in Figure 2).

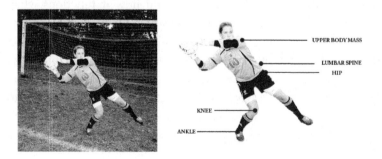

Figure 2. The vulnerability of the body's weak link in the presence of core stability deficits. In this instance, the knee is the weakest link, and

it collapses inward from lack of core control (especially in the glutes, which function to keep your knee in proper alignment with your hip and ankle).

Under static conditions, like when you're standing still, weakened core control may not result in any significant injurious forces or displacements. However, under dynamic conditions, like when you're jumping or running, your body will be subjected to much greater forces and displacements, and if you have poor core control, you'll be far more susceptible to injury. This is why injuries occur in dynamic conditions much more often than in static conditions (although you may only notice an injury once you're sitting down and begin to feel pain).

Your core generates stability and propulsive force throughout all of your movements, such as reaching, throwing, walking, running, going up or down stairs, squatting, and jumping. Without core stability, you get too much movement in other joints of your body's chain, like a wave of dominos falling. For example, a runner with poor core stability will have excessive movement in the pelvis, which may cause hip pain and damage. This also puts strain on the band of connective tissue that runs from your hip to your knee along the outside of your thigh. Over time, this may cause an overuse problem called IT (iliotibial) band syndrome. This tightness affects the kneecap's normal path of movement in relation to your other bones, and leads to other common painful injuries, such as patella-femoral syndrome (inflammation and pain in the front of the knee). The excessive movement of your leg can also lead to shin splints, or foot problems such as plantar fasciitis and other stubborn, painful injuries.

Core stability provides the foundation from which power is generated during cycling and promotes improved alignment throughout the body's chain, reducing risk of injury. While riding, a stable core prevents slumping and twisting of the trunk, which compromises biomechanics and saps power from the pedal stroke. A weak or fatigued core causes excessive and inefficient motion of the whole body, with more side-to-side motion instead of straight plane, piston motion. This not only wastes energy, but compromises performance and wreaks havoc on your back, hips, knees, ankles, and feet.

Fortunately, you have the power to reduce the risk of mishaps and injuries like those noted above by building your core stability, which is also important for your upper body. The scapulae, commonly known as the shoulder blades, are the large, flat wing bones that sit on your rib cage in your upper back. Like your kneecaps, your shoulder blades do not directly connect to the rest of your bones, and thus rely on the coordination of your core muscles for control. If these muscles are not working together in a coordinated manner to stabilize the shoulder blade, you can develop problems throughout your arm, including the shoulder, elbow, wrist, and hand. Upper body strength and stability rely heavily on the strength of your core foundation, just as a tree relies on the strength of its roots. It doesn't matter how strong the top branches are, if what's beneath them can't provide enough support. Weakness in the larger, stronger muscles of your core can cause altered biomechanics, overuse, pain, and injury in the smaller muscles further down your arm, such as tennis elbow, golfer's elbow, and even tendonitis in your hand.

These examples are just a few of the many negative consequences that can occur when your core does not stabilize your kinetic chain, putting all parts of your body at risk of injury. The good news is that you can train your core and create good biomechanics throughout your body to avoid painful injuries from head to toe.

Open vs. Closed Kinetic Chain for Your Core

"Life is your teacher, and you are in a state of constant learning."
—Bruce Lee

You may have heard the terms "open" and "closed" kinetic chain exercise at the gym or in a fitness blog, but what exactly do these terms mean and why are they important concepts for your core? To understand these terms, begin by thinking of the movements you perform in your daily life.

Your body's chain is considered open when the part you're moving is free in space, and not resting on a surface such as the ground, the wall, a tabletop, or the platform of a weight machine. Examples of open chain activities are waving your hand or lifting your leg, because they engage primarily the muscles directly involved in the movement of that body part. Open chain exercises are great for improving strength and function in isolation. This can help you become more aware of the specific muscles being used. Think of a bodybuilder with big guns formed from bicep curls, bulging quads from seated leg extensions, and six-pack abs from crunches. Yet, open chain exercises do not provide balanced and functional strength to control your kinetic chain across multiple joints, which is necessary for a healthy body. That's why you also need closed chain exercises.

In closed chain activities and exercises, the hand or foot is fixed with constant contact to an immobile surface. These exercises are the best way for you to achieve a healthy, functioning core and body. During closed chain activities, multiple segments of your body contract at the same time to stabilize and control movements across multiple joints. Closed chain exercises, such as push-ups, pull-ups, squats, leg presses, and lunges, are more functional because they train your muscles in ways that mimic the movements you make in real life and sports.

Generating Core Force

"Just as ripples spread out when a single pebble is dropped into water, the actions of individuals can have far-reaching effects."
—Dalai Lama

Want to throw a ball farther, run faster, or spike a volleyball harder? You can do all of these things by learning to control your core better. Your core is the most powerful part of your entire kinetic chain when it comes to generating force, and you can prove this to yourself in under sixty seconds. Try throwing a ball as far as you can without moving your trunk, and take note of how far it goes. Then, throw it again by cocking your arm and twisting your body backwards like a pitcher or quarterback, then stepping forward and pivoting at your hips as you bring your arm forward to release the ball. At least 50 percent more energy and force, developed in your lower body and trunk, will be funneled through the arm. Not only will the ball travel farther and faster when you use your core, but you will be putting less strain on the muscles of your arm and shoulder by employing more of your trunk's strength. This exercise shows that if you use your core appropriately, you'll generate significantly more power and greatly reduce your risk of injury at the same time!

Merely strengthening your pitching arm or kicking leg will not give you the performance enhancement you are looking for. My patient, Luke, is a star college baseball pitcher who learned this the hard way. Throughout his years of pitching since little league, he was focused on strengthening his shoulder muscles. He was plagued by recurrent shoulder tendonitis, causing him to miss many games for rest and recuperation. It was only after he tore two of the tendons in his shoulder and had surgical repair that I met him to help him rehabilitate and get back in the game. Once he started adding core training to his workout, he finally achieved the 90 mph pitch he had always strived for, while also improving his throwing accuracy and increasing his sprinting speed—all after a serious injury and surgery! Luke not only improved his performance with core training, but also reduced strain on his shoulder and remained injury-free for the rest of his pitching career. Unfortunately, many coaches, trainers, and athletes still don't understand the importance of core training, so too many athletes fall short of their athletic potential and suffer from injuries that could have been prevented using the techniques you'll learn in this book.

To understand this concept of force generation and transmission from and through the core, imagine your body as a chain with interconnected links. To keep it simple, think of your arms as one link, the legs as another, and the core as the central link. A pitcher winds up to throw like a drawn-back catapult, with his core as the middle of the catapult. When he extends his trunk backwards, he is loading his core muscles and harnessing energy to be released as his trunk and arm come forward, creating more velocity and force. This same concept applies to all daily activities and sports. For instance, when serving a tennis ball, spiking a volleyball, or powering through the water, you bring your arm back and extend your trunk with a controlled eccentric, or lengthening, contraction to maximize the force generated when you drive your arm forward. It's like you are winding your body into a tight spring to unleash more power.

In order to understand how the body creates forces and motions throughout all of its segments, let's consider a bar suspended on a pivot, like a seesaw. A force acting on one side of the bar will cause the bar to rotate on a pivot, like when your partner on the seesaw goes up as your force pulls your side down. The rotational motion that is produced (how hard and fast your partner goes up in the air) depends on the size of the force (how heavy you are) and the distance from the pivot point (the arm, or how far you are sitting from the middle).

This is what physicists and biomechanists refer to as "torque" when describing muscles that act on joints.

For the bar (or seesaw or joint) to remain stable, the torque on one side of the pivot point must be balanced by the torque on the other side. So, when a person holds a cup of coffee in their hand, the weight of the coffee cup leads to a torque acting on the pivot point (the wrist). This torque must be balanced by the lower arm, which in turn creates a torque on the next pivot point (the elbow). The torque from the lower arm must be balanced by the upper arm, and in turn, the upper arm creates a torque on the shoulder that must be balanced by your core.

That's why lifting a heavy load without proper core stabilization to counteract the torque that has moved through your body's chain can lead to a back injury. Regardless of where motion starts, whether you are picking up a bucket of water with your hand or kicking a soccer ball with your foot, movement and forces ripple upwards and downwards to adjoining links of your chain. You need lots of torque to throw a ball, make a fast movement, or move a heavy weight, but you must also be able to balance the torque, or face the damage done to the weakest links in your kinetic chain.

Here's another great analogy: Imagine throwing a pebble into a pond. The pebble makes a ripple that moves away from where it landed. As the pebble falls deeper into the pond, the water near the surface rushes back to fill in the space it left behind, causing a splash—the bigger the pebble, the bigger the splash. The splash then creates even more ripples that move outward from where it first landed in the water.

When water is in its calmest, lowest-energy state, it has a flat surface. By throwing the pebble into the pond, you have given the water some kinetic energy. That causes the water to move around, as it tries to spread around the energy and return to its still, flat state. The ripples that you see in the pond are small waves carrying away the energy from where you threw the pebble. Energy cannot be destroyed and will travel infinitely if it is not absorbed, just like when black holes collide and their violent union sends shock waves through space and time that can be detected billions of light years away. Your core is just like the crashing stone, or the colliding black holes. It's what creates the rings of energy that start in the center of your body, and then expands the ripple of energy outwards to the periphery of your body.

Your core is also what stops the energy once you've completed your movement. Remember, energy will travel infinitely if it's not absorbed, and your core muscles are your most important shock absorbers. Your core must be really good at resisting and stopping movement. Think of a football player running a pattern, stopping on a dime to fake out his opponent, and then cutting across the field. During the quick change of direction, the core is resisting the force of inertia that wants to continue to pull the receiver forward in motion. Core activation resists and prevents the receiver's trunk from toppling forward, and transfers force and movement when changing directions quickly to prevent injury and maximize performance.

Without a stable core, your limbs will not function optimally, and power will be sapped from all of your movements, leaving you more susceptible to falls and injuries. It is true that every link in a chain is important, but your core is the biggest, strongest, and most important central link that protects your body from injury. Learning to use your core better will allow you to generate more power and improve your performance in any physical activity. In almost every physical therapy patient I've seen, core training is the missing link in their overall fitness, whether they're an elite athlete or someone trying to recover from a nagging injury.

Seeds for Thought

- Until now, which muscles or areas of your body have you focused on most in your workouts?

- Do you feel your core muscles contracting (concentrically, eccentrically, and isometrically) throughout your day?

- When you did your self-assessment in the mirror, what did you notice about your posture? Where did you find imbalances (if any)?

- Have you tried "switch hitting" to balance asymmetries during daily activities with your non-dominant side?

- Are there any activities you'd like to improve your overall strength and performance in? Are you beginning to see how better control of your core muscles will help improve your performance?

CHAPTER 3

How Does Your Core Stack Up?

> "Respect the building blocks, master the fundamentals, and the
> potential is unlimited."
> —P.J. Ladd

Just like a tower of building blocks, the human body needs a strong foundation to be stable. Without a stable core, you may experience fatigue, weakness, pain, or trouble with balance, coordination, and performance. After their first faceplant off a skateboard, or watching a tower of blocks come crashing down, a child learns at a young age about the powerful force of gravity. As we grow older, we start to consider gravity the enemy as we fight for firm skin, a toned body, and a life without injury.

The Core BASE Guide will re-acquaint you with this monumental force of nature as your friend. You will learn to reap the benefits of Mother Earth's natural force on your body, starting with your ABC's: alignment, breathing, and core muscle function (which includes activation, strength, timing, and endurance). These fundamental building blocks will set you up for a strong, sound, and stable structure that won't crash. Instead, you'll improve your balance and help prevent osteoporosis, which 200 million people suffer from worldwide.

The foundation for core training begins with strong, natural postural alignment and optimal core muscle activation, which go hand in hand. Optimal core muscle function is dependent upon good posture (maintaining your spine's three innate curves in a neutral position), and good posture is dependent on optimal core function. Poor posture and poor core muscle activation are the main contributing factors that cause angry backs, necks, shoulders, hands, and knees, as well as compromised circulation and chronic fatigue. During activity your core muscles become fatigued and have a harder time providing the proper support your spine needs, which compromises your posture and control, thus lowering the threshold it takes to damage or injure your spine.

Back pain is one of the leading causes of disability around the world. Most people suffer at least one debilitating episode of pain in their spines at some point in their lives. Many of us have common abnormalities in our spines such as arthritis and degeneration, bulging, herniation, or disc extrusion, which may cause pain in some people, but not others. An MRI (magnetic resonance imaging) may not only be a waste of time and money, but having one of these tests may actually make things worse, because when you start to look for abnormalities, you will find them. Studies show that more than half of asymptomatic people have bulging discs in their spines. I actually have two extruded discs (completely blown out) in my neck from wiping out on my mountain bike, but I am happy to say I have no pain. Bed rest, pain medicine, injections, and surgery are often ineffective, and may leave you with an even angrier back that has given up and forgotten how to function in life.

Unfortunately, doctors all over the world still prescribe bed rest, even though it is the worst thing you can do. "If it hurts, don't do that!" advice will alleviate what is triggering your pain, and temporarily decrease your symptoms, but this is not the solution. If the source of your pain is not specifically addressed, your pain will eventually come back. Recent studies show that when young, healthy volunteers spent weeks in bed, their inner core muscles wasted away and forgot how to activate, taking months to recover. Eliminating the postural stressors that caused your symptoms in the first place and training your core to become balanced and resilient to injury are what really matter.

Unhealthy lifestyle factors cause a lot of painful backs. Obesity, which is an issue for 70 percent of Americans, causes pain-triggering inflammation and puts mechanical strain on the spine and discs, which causes neck, back, arm, and leg pain, as well as numbness, tingling, burning, and paralysis. Smoking is also a major risk factor for back pain because it clogs and damages the blood vessels that nourish your spine, leading to muscle and bone deterioration. Research clearly shows that sitting and slumping puts stress on the core muscles, ligaments, and discs that support the spine. This, in turn, weakens the core muscles that promote good posture and back health.

Spinal Architecture for Your Core Foundation

"Architecture is really about well-being."
—Zaha Hadid

For optimal core mechanics, the spine should be perfectly aligned vertically, with your entire body in a straight line from head to toe. When standing in good posture, or natural, neutral alignment, your chin should be parallel to the floor, shoulders even, and arms at your sides, with your body weight evenly distributed on both legs. "Standing up straight" is actually "standing up curved," allowing for your three distinct natural curves of your spine, in the shape of a stretched out "S." Without this "S" shape, the vertebrae would be completely straight up and down, which would subject your spine to tremendous wear and tear from vibration and impact, and limit the spring-like action of your spine as a shock-absorber.

From a side view your neck should be curved inward, with your mid back curved outward, and your lower back curved inward for optimal core alignment (Figure 3). Your ribs should be directly over your hips, and your butt should be gently lifted, not tucked. By slightly lifting your butt, you will tilt your pelvis slightly forward, which supports your lower back curve. This natural neutral posture is the most efficient position for flexibility, movement, stability, and protection from potentially injurious stressors.

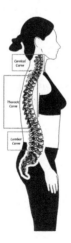

Figure 3. Good postural alignment, maintaining the three natural curves of the spine (cervical, thoracic, and lumbar) for optimal breathing and core functioning.

Developing Awareness of Your Own Core Alignment

"It is through the alignment of the body that I discovered the
alignment of the mind, self and intelligence."
—B.K.S Iyengar

Stand with your back against a wall, with your heels six inches
from the wall. Imagine balancing a cup of tea on your head. Take a deep
breath in and grow tall by lengthening your spine through the crown
of your head and lifting your ears away from your shoulders. Simply
standing up a little taller will automatically engage and tone your core.
Place your hands on your hips and note the expansion between your
fingers as you rise toward the sky. Using your hand, check the distance
between your neck and the wall. Push your head straight back against
the wall, making sure not to raise your chin up or down. If there is
significant space behind your head, place a rolled-up towel or pillow
behind it to push back into. As you push your head back, your trunk
should slide away from the wall until your shoulders line up with
your ears. Strive to keep this distance between your neck and the wall
under two inches and note how this feels. Try to maintain this position
throughout the day and track your progress by performing this self-
assessment often. You will be surprised how quickly you can correct
your posture once you develop core awareness.

Fix Your Couch Slouch

"Sitting still is a pain in the ass."
—Noah Levine

American adults sit for an average of six and a half hours per day,
while children sit for an average of eight hours per day, so it's important
to stay comfortable and aligned. Sitting with good postural alignment is
also critical for optimizing core muscle activation for postural support.
There should be 90-degree angles at your ankles, knees, hips, and
elbows, and a straight vertical line from the top of the head through
your hips (Figure 4). If your seat height is not adjustable, try using a
footstool or pad to maintain these right angles. When working on a

computer, position your screen so that the top is at your eye level. Your eyeline will then fall slightly below this, at approximately nose-level on the screen. The screen should be about eighteen inches from your face, and it should also be slightly tilted so the bottom is coming toward you, angled 10–20 degrees. Whenever possible, use a supportive pillow behind your lower back to reinforce your lower spine's natural forward curve, and to maintain alignment of the spinal segments above.

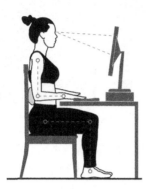

Figure 4. Ideal postural alignment while sitting, maintaining the three natural curves of the spine for optimal breath and core function.

Slumped, rounded posture may be avoided by keeping your shoulders down and slightly back, and opening up your chest by imagining your clavicles, or collarbones, "smiling." "Smiling" is accomplished by widening these two long, S-shaped bones at the top front of your chest, on either side of your sternum (or breastbone) (Figure 5). It is important to not over-clench the muscles in your mid-back, as this will limit the expansion in your back ribs. Imagine spreading your wings by allowing the bottoms of your shoulder blades to spread apart, and keep the back of your trunk spacious while opening your chest. This allows you to create space in your chest and simultaneously open up your ribcage in all directions. The ribcage must expand for optimal activation of the core stabilizing musculature that will pull you out of your slump. This activation is important for maintaining the critical tension needed to progress to core empowerment.

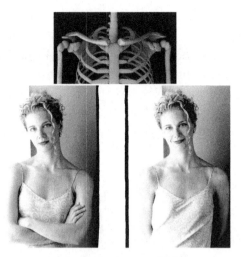

Photograph © Benjamin Dimmitt

Figure 5. Spread your wings with wide, "smiling" collarbones, illustrated by the image to the right. Compare this to the left image with rounded shoulders.

Good core alignment reduces pain, boosts muscle health, and decreases fatigue while improving your breathing, circulation, digestion, concentration, body image, and postural muscle strength. Recent evidence supports the bidirectional relationship between your core alignment and your emotional and spiritual state. Your physical stance, or the way you carry yourself, influences your physiology, emotions, and attitude. Open your heart and chest, staying mindful of your posture throughout the day and elongating your spine to encourage alertness and confidence. Do this while you are brushing your teeth, working at your desk, walking, or cooking to stay prepared for whatever challenge comes your way, both physically and emotionally.

Static Posture = Position / Dynamic Alignment = Action

"Human beings are
soft and supple when alive,
stiff and straight when dead.
The myriad creatures, the grasses and the trees are
soft and fragile when alive,
dry and withered when dead.
Therefore, it is said:

The rigid person is a disciple of death;
the soft, supple, and delicate are lovers of life.

An army that is inflexible will not conquer;
a tree that is inflexible will snap.
The unyielding and mighty shall be brought low;
The soft supple, and delicate will be set above."
—Lao Tzu

Optimal posture is achieved when the spine is upright with each vertebra stacked like building blocks that form a structure in a static, or non-moving, position. If the orientation of the blocks is not structurally sound, any sort of disturbance will cause the entire structure to come tumbling down. The vertical references for ideal postural alignment are helpful for identifying muscular and structural imbalances.

However, you also need to develop your own awareness of when your core is not reflecting good posture. You need this awareness to activate your trunk muscles and make the appropriate changes in your body's position for dynamic stability. Each time you make a correction, you are training your core. Over time, your core will get used to being in a good posture, and maintaining this posture will become a habit instead of a chore.

Your body is a dynamic system that can stretch, twist, and bend in three dimensions. Good dynamic alignment, or postural control, refers to the constantly shifting adjustments your core makes in relation to the rest of your body and the forces from the world around you. Struggling to maintain a static posture for prolonged periods may be a strenuous, frustrating endeavor that can leave you feeling fatigued, tense, stiff, sore, and grouchy. Sitting or standing up perfectly straight like a stack of blocks can also be exhausting. Instead, strive for graceful, fluid alignment in all your daily activities and athletic endeavors, so that your body's energy exerts an upward force to balance what's pulling you down.

Move and change your position as often as possible, while always gravitating toward your optimal alignment as your state of equilibrium. This will take conscious effort at first, but with time it will become second nature, preventing muscle fatigue, promoting circulation in your spine, and alleviating tension in your muscles, joints, and spirit.

If you feel antsy when you have to sit for a long period of time, that's normal. You should listen to your body's urges to move and stretch your muscles.

If you have to sit for more than thirty minutes, put some motion in your ocean by doing shoulder or trunk circles. Sitting for prolonged periods without movement, or "tucking your tailbone," shortens your hip flexors (the iliopsoas muscle group). This muscle group is located deep on both sides of the lower abdomen and includes the smaller iliacus (which connects the pelvis with the thigh) and the bigger psoas (which connects the spine with the thigh) (Figure 6). Due to a new understanding of the important role these muscles play, the psoas muscles have received a lot of attention lately not just as hip flexors, but also as stabilizers of your core, breath, and spirit.

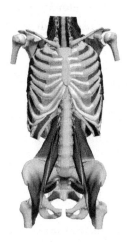

Figure 6. Your psoas and quadratus lumborum muscles are important deep core stabilizers that provide structural support to each side of your spine, like "guy-wires" or violin strings. Source: Medical Historical Library, Harvey Cushing/John Hay Whitney Medical Library, Yale University.

This pair of core-stabilizing muscles is unique, as they are the only ones in your body that connect your legs to your spine, with connections to your diaphragm, core floor, and the fight or flight response of your nervous system. Chronic tension in these muscles may cause back, hip, or knee pain, as well as inefficient breathing, digestive problems, and anxiety. It can also cause your belly to protrude. Prolonged positioning in flexion shortens your psoas muscles and leads to twinging backs. This is caused by a tug of war between your psoas muscles that pulls on the front of your spine to flex it, and the quadratus lumborum muscles that pulls on the back of the spine to restore your natural alignment.

Relieve this tension by placing a rolled towel, cushion, or wedge in your chair to adjust the position of your pelvis. Adjusting your position, sitting on a ball, or taking frequent breaks to stand and move will release the tension in your psoas muscles, diaphragm, pelvic floor, and mind, helping to prevent structural and emotional imbalances.

Get up and walk as often as possible to stretch your tight psoas and wake up your sleepy butt. When you walk, you are naturally stretching out your psoas in the leg that is trailing behind, and you can get even more stretch by making sure the heel of this back leg stays in contact with the ground without lifting up. Focus on quieting your steps, which requires stronger activation of your posterior chain. Engaging and tightening your glutes actually helps to relax your psoas through what is called "reciprocal inhibition," which is when muscles on one side of a joint relax to accommodate contraction on the other side. Each heel strike will increase your posterior chain tone, stretch out your tight hip flexors, and give you a little more pep in your step!

Studies show that people who switch to standing desks feel significantly less back pain. When you're standing at your desk, or in general, try shifting your weight from one foot to the other to feel the movement in your hips and core to help you improve your dynamic alignment, core stability, and blood flow.

Sleep posture is also important for your core and overall health. We spend roughly one third of our lives sleeping to replenish our mind-body-spirit. During the day, as you are up and about, the nourishing fluid in your spinal discs seeps out due to the effects of gravity. While you sleep, your discs in between your vertebrae fill with fluids that lubricate, nourish, and lengthen your spine, actually making you "grow" about a half inch in your sleep. Make sure your mattress is firm enough to give your spine good support. Avoid using more than one small pillow for your head, as this will cause strain on your spine and contribute to a forward head posture. Choose one that allows you to maintain your head and spine in your neutral position with your natural, curved alignment. Learn to sleep on your back or your side instead of on your belly, which causes strain on your neck and compromises the blood flow to your brain. Placing a second small pillow under your knees while lying on your back (or between your knees when on your side) may help to position your spine with its natural curves.

Poor alignment is indicative of a weak, ineffective core, and hinders the ability to take a deep, nourishing breath. This lack of proper breathing and alignment can inhibit proper stretching or activation of the inner core muscles, thus compromising core stability. This is particularly important when bending and lifting, as such activities put more pressure on your back.

When you lift a heavy object, you should hinge at your hips with your knees slightly bent, keeping your spine in its natural, neutral position, rather than arching or rounding the back, which puts you at greater risk of injury. Hip hinging wakes up your core muscles and protects the joints of your spine and legs. With practice, this movement will provide the functional foundation for day-to-day movements like bending over your sink or getting in your car, or more complex movements in sports, such as spiking a volleyball. Good alignment puts your core musculature in optimal position for deep, nourishing breathing and optimal core muscle activation to establish your Core BASE for safe and powerful movement.

Sense Your Core Alignment

"A good stance and posture reflect a proper state of mind."
—Morihei Ueshiba

Awareness of your core is learned through two different proprioceptive pathways. I have learned from our studies that it is important to consider both of these aspects of proprioception, or your "sixth sense." You can learn to sense your core alignment through your static and dynamic proprioceptors. These special cells are located in all the joints of your body. Static proprioceptors allow you to sense the position of your joints, whereas dynamic proprioceptors give you awareness of joint movement.

Static Core Posture: Stand with your feet hip-width apart, close your eyes, and try to maintain a completely still position. Notice how difficult it is to not move, what happens to your breath, and how your trunk muscles feel as you attempt to stay motionless. Do your core muscles stiffen so much that you compromise your body's natural ability to adjust, move, or breathe deeply? Your static proprioceptors will eventually start screaming at your muscles, creating tension, soreness, and pain to the point that your muscles just give up and succumb to a slouch.

Dynamic Core Alignment: Now stand up and move around for a minute or two, then slowly tune back in to your breath and lengthen your naturally curved spine. Keep your eyes closed and relax your muscles just enough to keep yourself from tipping over. Allow yourself to gracefully shift your weight as needed to maintain your position. Listen to your body, and you will find that you naturally experience some swaying and correction. Your core is adjusting to changes in your body and your environment. Notice how you breathe more deeply and feel more stable, centered, and energized when you are not forcing stillness.

Focus less on maintaining static rigid posture and more on dynamic core alignment to stabilize your body without compromising your breath or creating muscle tension and stiffness. Some of my colleagues refer to "stiffness" in their publications as a good thing, but I think that term may be a bit confusing. When loads are placed on the core muscles, they contract; when the core muscles contract, they create stiffness. Stiffness is an important component of injury prevention because it prevents your spine from buckling under a load. Yet, as in the parable of the oak and reed, the oak tree is stiffer but snaps, whereas the reed is less stiff, but able to bounce back. True core stability is the ability to react at the right time with the right amount of stiffness.

Core alignment is a full-body experience, and your body is designed for mobility. Think of a surfer's trunk shifting in all directions to respond to the waves, or a boxer who dances around his opponent to avoid a punch. Both athletes are dynamically stable as their cores are moving, and they maintain control of their body's center of gravity. So, hang loose and fly like a butterfly to withstand all the perturbations and punches life brings your way with a fluid, adaptable, and dynamically stable core.

Pandiculation: Nature's Way of Aligning Your Core

"By discovering nature, you discover yourself."
—Maxime Lagace

If you watch your furry pet wake up from its rest, you'll see that they naturally arch their backs, then reverse the motion and drop to their bellies to curve downward, lengthening the legs, back, and belly in a full body yawn. Moving back and forth between extreme positions of the spine helps to reset their alignment before they run off to play. This is called pandiculation, and it is something we have naturally been doing for millions of years to relax tight, tense muscles.

From prolonged positioning, your muscles learn to stay in suboptimal positions, where some muscles are contracted in a shortened position, and the opposing muscles are stretched or lengthened. These compromised muscle lengths become set in your brain, nerves, and the position sensors of your body, putting your body in an unbalanced auto-pilot mode. Pandiculation is a way to reset your body's software and reboot your sensation and muscle control to their optimal functioning lengths.

As humans, we pandiculate even before we are born, as revealed by imaging studies and the magical kicking mothers feel from their unborn babies. We naturally want to pandiculate upon waking, as we gently tighten our jaws, arms, and legs before yawning, then reach our arms overhead as we stretch our legs out. When we do this, we are first contracting our muscles, then slowly lengthening them, and finally relaxing. This natural sequential pattern allows our brains to integrate the new feedback, resetting our muscle lengths and alignment. Alternately contracting and releasing will decrease the tension on your muscles and nerves.

Pandiculation also improves proprioception, because when you contract a muscle, your brain (the command center of your muscles) receives sensory feedback and responds with renewed voluntary muscle control, coordination, and relaxation. Your nervous system learns through awareness of your movement to release accumulated tension. Improved neural connections not only help the way you move, but also improve the way you think. So next time you want to stretch, try first contracting the muscle that's tight, slowly lengthening it, then completely relaxing. Note the difference not only in sensation and control of the muscle, but also in your range of motion and sense of ease throughout your body.

In our modern, fast-paced lives, many people have become sedentary and stressed through much of their days. As creatures of habit, we find ourselves maintaining the same postures for long periods of time, as we get so caught up in our higher cognitive functioning that we forget about our innate, primitive instinct to align our bodies. Get back in touch with your primitive animal spirit and pop some pandiculation into your day for an innate technique that will release muscular and emotional tension, reduce pain, increase mobility, and improve your posture and core alignment for optimal functioning.

Transform Your Vicious Cycle into a Virtuous Cycle

"Some people drive themselves into a vicious cycle. There is always a way out; a delightful inner opening."
—Tina Panossian

Your core muscles work best if your body is in good postural alignment. A vicious cycle occurs when poor posture creates weakness and imbalance of your core muscles, because this causes your core muscles to work less efficiently, requiring more energy and force to move, and further compromising your posture. Conversely, the better your core alignment, the more efficient and stable your core will be, which in turn reinforces good alignment throughout your body. Good posture also improves your breathing mechanics (which also improves your core muscle efficiency).

Start your day with perfect poise and remind yourself to continuously correct your alignment throughout the day, whether you are tapping your keyboard, driving a truck, or sitting in front of your TV. Stress, fatigue, and gravity cause you to shrug and slump your shoulders, protrude your chin forward, round your mid back like a turtle, and collapse your lower back on your butt, causing your belly to push out.

Cultivating good posture will help you stand taller, look slimmer, and find your grace against gravity.

Seeds for Thought

- What did you observe about your core alignment?

- If you noticed that you were out of your natural, optimal alignment, practice using your core awareness to adjust and correct your posture.

- On average, how much time do you spend seated each day? Can you make it a habit to maintain better core alignment when you sit?

- Can you think of any solutions you could implement to reduce the time you spend sitting consecutively, or to take more frequent breaks to stand and move your body?

- How does it feel to practice proper posture? Do you notice any effects on your breathing, comfort and mindset?

CHAPTER 4

How Your Sex Impacts Your Core Health and Injury Risk

"Challenges are gifts that force us to search for a new center of gravity."
—Oprah Winfrey

From her birth in western Ukraine in 1938, my mother grew to be a brave, resilient, and intellectually curious girl. The ninth of ten children born to a schoolmistress mother and Ukrainian Catholic priest father, she survived the war, witnessed Nazi atrocities in her village of Brody, fled with her family by horse-drawn cart over the mountains to Slovakia to escape the Soviet army (they were rounding up and killing Ukrainian Catholic priests at the time), experienced bombs overhead in Vienna, and spent months in refugee camps in Bavaria before emigrating to Canada. Of all these traumatic childhood memories, the one that she remembered most clearly was a fall she suffered while secretly attempting to ride her brother's bicycle. The laceration on her chin was secondary to the pain she felt when her father severely scolded her for "unfeminine" behavior, as girls were not allowed to venture outside the confines of traditional female roles (such as cooking, cleaning, sewing, and embroidering clothes to dress up pretty on Sundays and holidays).

My mother shared this story with me in the late 1970s, when I came home from school in tears after being disciplined for playing soccer with the boys at recess, which was still strictly forbidden. Title IX had already been enacted, which opened the door for girls to participate more in sports, but in my small Ukrainian Catholic school in Western New York, these changes were slow to come. Despite this, my mother encouraged me to join the boys' soccer team at school (since we didn't have a girls' team), play all the rough sports my brothers and cousins played, and race them on foot, in water, or on bicycles. She told me if I tried hard enough, I could do anything they could.

Looking back, this was rather progressive thinking for a time when most mothers were more worried about potential injuries blemishing their daughter's beauty. Today, a scar on my chin from my own bicycle fall, almost identical to my mother's, always reminds me of her strength and encouragement to challenge traditional gender roles. As opportunities for girls and women have increased, the concept of beauty has also dramatically evolved, and today its definition is more inclusive than ever, recognizing our bodies, minds, and spirits.

Since the inception of Title IX in 1972, there has been a ten-fold increase in female sports participation, which has provided girls with tremendous physical, psychological and spiritual benefits. However, the dramatic increase in the number of girls and women playing sports, combined with their greater susceptibility to injury compared to boys and men, has resulted in an epidemic of female injuries that have tremendous physical, emotional, and financial repercussions. There are several reasons for the dramatic differences in injury rates between the sexes: anatomical, hormonal, neuromuscular, psychological, and genetic, each of which I will describe in detail. Understanding these factors and knowing which ones we can influence with experience and training is key to preventing injuries and promoting overall healthy functioning of the human body.

Sex-Based Differences of Injury Mechanisms

"Our greatest glory is not in never falling, but in rising every time
we fall."
—Confucius

I sustained a high-force injury after presenting my research at the 1st World Congress for Injury Prevention in Oslo, Norway. While mountain biking on the majestic fjords, I fell fifty feet down a steep, rocky cliff. So why is it that I survived with only minor injuries despite such high forces acting upon my body, whereas another woman may sustain incapacitating lifelong injuries from a slip in the shower (a relatively minor event with much lower destabilizing forces)? Because different women have different levels of proprioception and core control, and it's these two factors that play the largest role in injury prevention. My scientific research shows that females activate their core musculature differently from males when performing dynamic activities, with less core posterior chain activation and less control of their trunks, which makes them move their bodies differently and increases their risk of injury. You can find a video demonstration of these differences at www.doczaz.com.

My colleagues have extensively studied differences in injury mechanisms between the sexes by reviewing thousands of hours of video analysis and computer modeling. They determined that while male injuries are predominantly contact injuries (such as sports collisions), female injuries are usually non-contact in nature and involve a loss of control of the center of mass outside the base of support, rendering the weak link in the body's chain susceptible to injury. Non-contact injuries are likely to happen during deceleration and acceleration motions (such as a quick change in direction to avoid an oncoming opponent), with loss of trunk control. These same injury mechanisms are also found in men, but incidences of non-contact injuries and loss of trunk control are much higher in women.

Your body is made up of many interconnected segments that influence each other. Imbalanced forces and motions generated at one joint affect all of the remaining joints. Thus, problems in the control of one segment (or instability in the most extreme cases) may degrade the performance of the other segments to the point that the entire system may become unstable. Impaired proprioception, or impaired relay of this information through your nervous system, compromises dynamic core control. Accurate timing of core muscle activation and the right amount of core muscle strength are critical components of your body's ability to maintain stability, decrease your susceptibility to injury, and improve your ability to recover from injuries.

Anatomical Factors

"Nobody is superior, nobody is inferior, but nobody is equal either.
People are simply unique, incomparable."
—Osho

Due to the epidemic of female injuries that we've witnessed over the past forty years, scientists have been studying anatomical differences in body structure between the sexes, and how these differences relate to the higher injury rates in females compared with males. Much of this research has involved the study of musculoskeletal injuries in sports. This disparity, specifically related to body structure, has been attributed to intrinsic factors such as height, weight, body mass, body fat content, flexibility, loose ligaments, limb size, biomechanical alignment, and structural bone and joint differences that may be related to growth and maturation factors.

These disparities between females and males have been implicated and extensively researched, but no definitive correlation has been proven, thus rendering the influence of anatomical factors on higher injury rates in females inconclusive. The lack of consensus may stem from variability in baseline risk for different activities and sports, differences in objective measures of anatomical risk factors, inconsistency in methodology for classification of injuries, and the timing and frequency of data collection. Furthermore, structural anatomical factors are not easily modifiable, thus limiting the potential for intervention.

Young girls and boys do not exhibit different injury rates, but after puberty, when girls develop curves and a widening pelvis, the alignment of the pelvic floor in relationship to the rest of the body significantly changes, which changes the balance between muscles and creates injurious forces throughout the body. Mother Nature has an amazing ability to continue sculpting the female core from puberty through the childbearing years, whereas the male core anatomical structure remains the same throughout maturation. The female pelvis widens during reproductive years to accommodate the miracle of giving new life. Although you cannot change your structural anatomy, The Core BASE Guide will train your core to counteract and compensate for these changes, which will help to level the playing field between girls and boys and lower injury rates for both.

Women and men have anatomical differences in their reproductive systems that affect their abilities to stabilize their trunks and bodies during movement. Core training is particularly important for women because it can provide balance, strength, and stability to the muscles that bear the weight and trauma of pregnancy. This training can also lead to easier delivery and fewer complications post-partum, such as back pain, leg pain, and pelvic issues. Strategies to prevent these problems will be discussed in Chapter 6.

Hormonal Factors

"We cannot change anything until we accept it."
—Carl Jung

In order to understand how injury rate disparities can be leveled, it's important to first acknowledge inherent differences between the sexes. But why do these differences predispose women to suffer more injuries than men?

Scientists used to think that higher injury rates in women were related to hormonal differences. After the onset of puberty, girls and boys demonstrate differences in hormone levels, specifically in levels of estrogen, progesterone, and relaxin. Cyclical fluctuations of these hormones during the menstrual cycle have been hypothesized to affect the mechanical properties of ligaments and level of neuromuscular control (or lack thereof), thereby leading to disproportionately higher female injury rates. My colleagues and I have comprehensively studied these possible connections between hormones and injuries in females, and found that there is no sufficient evidence to support a direct hormonal influence on injuries in girls and women. What we did discover is that hormones may influence neuromuscular factors, such as proprioception, balance, and agility, and that these factors are the ones that predispose women to suffer more injuries.

This is very good news because proprioception, balance, and agility are all factors that you can significantly improve with training and practice, whereas controlling your hormone levels is much more difficult, and potentially quite dangerous. Although there is no conclusive evidence directly linking hormones to injury during a specific point in the menstrual cycle, it is important to realize that hormonal levels do create real effects on each of us individually. Hormone activity is considered by many medical professionals to be the fifth vital sign, making it just as important to your health as your heart rate, pulse, blood pressure, and temperature.

Hormones play a significant role in muscle development, which is crucial for core stability. Since women naturally have much lower levels of testosterone, and testosterone stimulates muscle growth, men tend to have more muscle mass than women. Less muscle mass, combined with more flexible joints in women, is a recipe for injury when joints are overloaded, which makes core training especially important for women. Core training also maximizes the benefits of high estrogen levels found in women during their reproductive years by building their bones to withstand the forces of everyday activities, as well as higher impact activities such as sports, while also protecting their bones from weakening and breaking as they grow older.

The cascade of hormones that rise and fall within women's bodies also affect their emotions, concentration, metabolism, coordination, dexterity, and performance. Women should develop awareness of their own hormonal fluctuations and specifically take note of how this affects them so they can use that information to reach their fullest potential. The United States women's soccer champions tracked their cycles and used this data to help them achieve peak performance on their road to victory, and every woman can do the same.

The team used comprehensive surveys of each of the twenty-three players, collecting information regarding the length of the players' periods, the symptoms they felt throughout their cycles, and how much and when the players felt their symptoms impacted their performance. This information was used to create an individualized profile for each athlete to determine practice duration and intensity for the weeks of the World Cup Tournament in France. Although these athletes used a sophisticated app, there are also free mobile apps that can track cycles and record symptoms. All women should monitor their cycles and symptoms to get in tune with their bodies as instruments they can learn to play to perfection!

Neuromuscular Factors

"The body is not a thing, it is a situation:
it is our grasp on the world and our sketch of our project."
—Simone de Beauvoir

Imagine a young girl who has just experienced a growth spurt, as some girls sprout as many as seven inches per year during puberty. Now, she has a bigger machine to manage with her existing motor programs, which are neuromuscular strategies that help her anticipate, plan, and guide her movements safely. As she matures, her upper body mass increases and adds proportionally more body fat than her male counterpart. Her core, and therefore her center of gravity, moves higher off the ground, figuratively putting her on stilts. Therefore, like balancing a broom stick with a weight on top, it is harder for her to control and balance her core compared to when she was prepubescent.

After their adolescent growth spurt, males experience a neuromuscular spurt, which involves rapid muscular development and proportionately more power compared to girls. Although boys acquire a bigger machine after a growth spurt, they also develop a proportionate neuromuscular engine, or powerhouse. After maturation, girls experience a heavier trunk and a center of mass located higher off the ground with their fat and lean body mass redistributed in novel ways, but they do not automatically develop a neuromuscular engine powerful enough to control that bigger machine as safely and effectively as boys do. The higher center of mass, combined with a wider pelvis, smaller and weaker muscles and bones, and looser ligaments, puts girls and women at greater risk for injury and pain throughout their bodies. Without targeted core muscle training, girls may not be able to overcome their potential biomechanical disadvantages.

To compound these biomechanical disadvantages, girls are now entering puberty about a year earlier than they did fifty years ago. The average age of breast development, which represents the first clinical sign of female puberty, has declined an average of three months per decade. The health implications of this shift are not fully clear, as there are still no long-term studies determining the implications of early breast development for women's lifelong health. However, early puberty in girls seems to be associated with a higher risk of obesity, diabetes, heart disease, and allergies.

There are several possible contributing factors to early puberty in girls. First, girls on average now have a higher body mass index (a measure of body fat based on height and weight) caused by excessive fat, and that fat tissue is related to the endocrine system, which produces and metabolizes hormones. These hormonal shifts may play a role in the earlier onset of puberty. Chemicals in the environment and in our diets may also be contributing factors, because many man-made chemicals are endocrine disruptors, or xenohormones, meaning they interact with the body's hormonal system in powerful and unintended ways.

Regardless of why girls are starting puberty sooner, it's clear that young girls today are confronted earlier in life with unique biomechanical challenges while trying to balance a higher center of mass, which subjects them to decreased neuromuscular control and possible injury. The best news is that both men and women can improve their neuromuscular control by using core training programs that develop the core engine to significantly decrease the prevalence of injuries.

Psychological Factors

"The reed that bends in the wind is stronger than the mighty oak which breaks in a storm."
—Confucius

Like my mother, my father also overcame much adversity throughout his childhood. In 1925, he was born in the quaint Ukrainian village of Komarno, only fifty miles from the future love of his life (my mother actually wasn't born yet, and they wouldn't meet until thirty years later in the Catskills of New York). Like most villages in Ukraine at that time, Komarno had been ravaged by the ugly realities of communism, and almost everyone there lived in severe poverty. My father was just seven years old when all of Ukraine began experiencing the horrific and devastating atrocity called Holodomor.

The Holodomor was an international genocide that took place between 1932 and 1933. During this time, Joseph Stalin and his Soviet regime deliberately starved millions of Ukrainian people to death for the purpose of crushing their will and desire for freedom and independence. The precise number of deaths has been debated by historians, but it is now reliably estimated to have been around ten million people, more deaths than the Jewish Holocaust. This brutal, ruthless, and savage evil forced my father to flee on his own to Western Europe just before his sixteenth birthday in 1941.

I can only imagine how agonizing it must have been to leave all he had known and travel across a continent afire with war, just for the chance to survive. In a great understatement, he once told me he felt relieved once he passed across the borders of the Soviet Empire, beyond the Iron Curtain. He said to himself, "Life will not be easy, but I survived," and sought to make the most of his life.

Not only did my father survive, but he thrived by developing a fierce determination, relentless self-reliance, and strong resilience that he would later instill in me as a young girl with the parable of the oak and the reed. The oak tree, although thicker and stronger, snaps and is blown over in the storm, whereas the reed bends in the wind and survives. Like the reed, my father's ability to adapt and persevere exemplifies a critical component of core resilience. As Bob Marley once said, "You never know how strong you are, until being strong is your only choice." Just as your core must grow resilient to perturbation, so must your spirit.

Each of us will experience adversity in our own turbulent times. The question is, how will you get through difficult times with non-negative thinking, and how can you learn and grow through perseverance and resilience? A pessimist focuses on the difficulty in every opportunity, whereas an optimist recognizes the opportunity in every difficulty. Negative experiences may be used to mobilize previously dormant potential from within. A tree hunkers down through the winter, yet grows bigger, stronger, and more beautiful when spring arrives. The scientific community is recognizing the importance of psychological attributes for wellness and injury prevention. Resilience, optimism, confidence, and positive self-perception are strong predictors of future wellness, and are skills that you can acquire and develop to improve your psychological outlook and prevent injury.

Females in particular have a higher risk of psychological contributors to injury due to hormonal and personality factors, as well as gender bias that still exists in athletics. For example, women are more likely to suffer from fear, anxiety, depression, insomnia, and eating disorders that may contribute to health issues and injuries. Yet, both men and women can benefit from effective strategies for improving mental health and wellness.

Meditation, yoga, Pilates, and martial arts have all been studied and shown to improve not just core stability, but also psychological factors that are important for health and injury prevention. In addition to strengthening the core, the benefits of these practices include reduced stress, decreased anxiety and depression, improved cognition, and reduced symptoms of chronic diseases, such as fibromyalgia (a medical condition characterized by chronic widespread pain) and lung disease.

Genetic Factors

"Genetics load the gun. Your lifestyle pulls the trigger."
—Dr. Mehmet Oz

The gap in injury occurrence between young women and men has recently been linked to the influence of genetics on the structure, function, and integrity of our ligaments. Tissue samples of torn ligaments from athletes after non-contact knee injuries revealed genes that give rise to specific proteins associated with ligament structure and strength. These genes were expressed differently in the ligaments from the females compared to those taken from the males.

These differences may account for the weaker anterior cruciate ligaments in injured females versus males, a conclusion which would have significant implications in athletics and sports medicine. This discovery may hopefully lead more young women to get genetic counseling prior to athletic participation, so those at higher risk and with need for specialized training can be identified. We can't change the x and y chromosomes that determine our sex, but we can help girls strengthen their cores with exercises and prevention programs proven to reduce injuries.

Genes are now recognized as key risk factors for athletic injuries. New research has shown that players with specific genotypes (types of DNA sequences) suffer from more ankle, knee, and total injuries, resulting in reduced sports participation. Genetic testing is now being used in professional sports to help identify athletes who are prone to injury to target them specifically for core neuromuscular training. Last year, China unveiled a plan to use genetic testing for performance and injury risk to aid in selection of its 2022 Olympic athletes.

Although new evidence indicates that our genes may predispose us to certain diseases, injuries, or outcomes, they do not solely determine our fate. Through exercise, psychological outlook, diet, and other lifestyle choices, you can actually change the way your DNA is expressed within your body to help you avoid injury, fight disease, and thrive. The research clearly shows that the choices you make every day will directly impact the expression of your genes and overall wellbeing, as well as that of your children. We are all created by DNA, but sculpted through our experiences from infancy. You'll learn more about how you can positively influence your genes with simple strategies and healthy lifestyle choices later in the book.

Natural Core Development

"By crawling, a child learns to stand."
—Danish Proverb

While men and women have inherent differences in hormones, anatomy, and other factors, there are steps that both can take to strengthen their cores and work their unique differences to their advantage. We can help new generations learn this as early as infancy, as babies are born with great joint mobility, but very little muscle control, and therefore little stability. As a baby grows, core control develops before coordinated, controlled arm and leg motions. The sequence of neuromuscular development begins on the belly, as the baby develops strength and control of the neck and back muscles by lifting its head against gravity, then progresses to abdominal muscle development while lying on the back. Next, the baby learns to sit by contracting all of its core muscles together. Only after this is core control achieved, and the infant may begin to use its arms for reaching, grasping, and changing positions. Generally, by one year of age, the baby has progressed to pulling upright and walking. This sequence of core muscle activity preceding muscle activity in the arms and legs is evident during all activities of daily life, as well as advanced upright activities, including standing, walking, running, jumping, and maneuvers of play.

When a child uses their tiny hand muscles to pick up a berry from the table and bring it to their mouth, they must have a stable chain of muscle activation running from the core to the elbow to the hand. If that chain of muscle activation beginning at the core isn't stable and strong, it will be difficult to get the berry to the target. This proximal strength and stability are required to support free movement in the distal body parts. Proximal stability is critical for distal mobility and athleticism.

"Proximal" and "distal" are anatomical terms used to describe how close or far a body part is from the core. Something proximal is closer to the core, whereas something distal is farther from the core. As the central reference point, the core is proximal, whereas the fingers and toes are the most distal segments of the body. Developmentally, all movement starts at our core. Central inner-core muscle pre-activation creates a stable foundation for distal movement of the arms and legs. This neuromuscular pattern of control has evolved in humans over millions of years and has resulted in the pure, natural, and efficient way we move today.

Core-stabilizing muscles are activated before your body initiates motion to control your spine. However, in people who have poor core muscle control, bad postural habits, and/or back pain, this natural activation of trunk muscles is reduced and delayed, meaning they turn on late, and with less strength. When this happens, the distal joints down the chain have to do extra work to stabilize, taking on a lot more force and becoming overworked, overstretched, or tight in an attempt to compensate, making your body's movements inefficient, unbalanced, and potentially injurious. To move properly and effectively, you must begin by training your core and your breath to restore the natural proximal to distal sequencing of your body's kinetic chain, which is developed during infancy to carry you through a lifetime of healthy movement and functioning.

Breathing and Core Stability

"The mind controls the body, but the breath controls the mind."
—B.K.S. Iyengar

On average, you take a breath every five seconds. That's twelve breaths a minute, 720 breaths per hour, 17,000 breaths each day, and over six million breaths per year, for a total of 500 million breaths in the average lifetime! If you want to optimize your daily activities and athletic performance, nourish your internal organs, and improve your overall health and functioning, it's important that you breathe efficiently, effectively, and effortlessly.

Healthy diaphragmatic breathing, or belly breathing, is an often-overlooked precursor and critical component of core stability. How does breathing help core stability? Simply put, if you cannot breathe deeply, you cannot brace your trunk properly, which means your body cannot function as it should. Your respiratory muscles work synergistically with your core muscles to achieve trunk control with subconscious, automatic stabilization. Practicing deep breathing increases activation and the size of your core stabilizing muscles, just like when you train your biceps with curls to get big arms. Breathing also has a powerful connection with your brain and mindset, and may automatically alter your state of mind by triggering neurons in your brain to tell your body it's time to calm down.

Deep, healthy breathing provides optimal oxygen input to your entire body. Lack of adequate blood flow compromises the oxygen supply and creates a cascade of events, including increased muscle tension, spasms, and pain, which adversely affect proprioceptive function and alter core muscle control and balance. This forces your body to rely more on distal or peripheral muscles and joints in order to compensate for loss of core stability, worsens peripheral muscle fatigue, and increases the load to your joints, thereby increasing your risk of injury. If you are not breathing deeply, not only is your back's function compromised because you are unable to brace properly, but so is the functioning of all parts of your body.

Newborns naturally breathe deeply, and ideally, they should continue deep breathing throughout their lives. Unfortunately, around age ten, most children begin to exhibit a pattern of shallow chest breathing, when the lungs do not fully expand, which compromises their core stability over time. As babies, we develop the innate knowledge of fully engaging the core for deep, refreshing breaths. As we grow older, due to mind and body stressors, we adapt a less efficient breathing method by shifting to a shallow pattern that deprives our bodies of the oxygen we need for healthy functioning, which also compromises the action of our core musculature. Chest breathing, which is common in preteens and teenagers, relies on muscles around your neck and collarbone instead of your core muscles, which causes fatigue, irritation, headaches, anxiety, increased muscle tension in the upper chest and shoulders, and decreased activation of essential core muscles.

In today's digital age, kids are sitting for long periods during the day, making it more difficult to fight the forces of gravity and maintain a strong, stable core. As children grow up, their posture also changes significantly due to a combination of factors, including chest development, rapid growth, and poorly balanced core muscles. Postural stance during those trying teenage years may be influenced by timidity due to new body composition, or sometimes adolescent rebellion. The weight of the world on their shoulders may contribute to a closed heart postural pattern, which demonstrates the self-protective posture where the chest sinks, the heart area collapses, and the upper spine and shoulders slump, further contributing to shallow breathing. When the chest breathing pattern is accompanied by poor posture, many muscles in the body aren't able to function properly because they become weak from being overstretched or tense from overuse.

Your nose is meant for breathing while your mouth is meant for drinking, eating, kissing, talking, singing, and laughing. Breathing through your mouth rather than your nose is another aberration that compromises respiratory function and contributes to a compensatory forward head posture. This creates musculoskeletal strain in the neck and may precipitate a cascade of negative events throughout your body. A forward head posture shifts your center of gravity forward and compromises core muscle function. Mouth breathing reduces oxygenation of your brain, heart, and all of your organs, which may cause infections and even learning disabilities, alter facial and dental growth, impair swallowing, create jaw problems, and affect sleep and overall quality of life. One quick thing you can do right now to begin improving your core strength and overall health is remind yourself to breathe through your nose and make sure your belly expands as you breathe in.

Poor posture not only interrupts healthy breathing patterns, but it also places your core musculature at a mechanical disadvantage. That's why people with poor posture experience more pain and functional impairment, which affects their wellbeing throughout life. Good posture optimizes efficient breathing, decreases wear and tear on the spine, trims your silhouette, and projects confidence. Parents and teachers must be educated regarding the importance of optimal spinal posture in growing children, as well as the recommendations you'll find later in the book for nurturing the natural core from infancy and helping timid turtles become proud peacocks!

Our bodies can survive weeks without food and days without water, but only moments without oxygen. The ageless wisdom of ancient breathing practices is inspiring a new consciousness in health and injury prevention, which is re-emerging in our medical culture. Connecting your core to the power of your breath drives health, athletic performance, and life.

Pre-activating Trunk Muscle Exercise

"Before anything else, preparation is the key to success."
—Alexander Graham Bell

Just as we all developed our core control before the control of our limbs as babies, we must re-learn this natural sequence of muscle activation for efficiency and effectiveness of all of our functional movements. Perform a simple exercise to help you feel the beneficial effects of pre-activating trunk muscles during activities. Position yourself in front of a chair with your legs hip-width apart and the back of your legs several inches in front of the chair. Without using your arms, slowly lower yourself down to a seated position. Then try the same task holding a five to ten-pound weighted object, with your arms out in front of you at chest height.

You should notice it's easier to control your descent and ascent back to standing position with the addition of the counterweight, which activates your trunk muscle prior to and during your movement. Feel for the firmness around your trunk with the added weight. If you can feel your core muscles activating, congratulations! You have a head start on your path to core empowerment. However, if you don't feel the muscle activation, no worries: you will develop this awareness as you continue practicing the Core BASE exercises.

This task demonstrates the importance of your core as the foundation for any purposeful movement of your body. Whether you are swinging a racket or vacuuming, the muscular force and control of motion originates at your center and travels through your limbs. A deficient core saps control and power from all movements of your body, whereas a stable core will allow greater ease and efficiency in everything you do and eliminate chaos and injury in the periphery.

Now imagine you are going to lift a heavier object, like a fifty-pound bag of dog food. With a stable core, you'll be able to maintain a neutral position of your trunk throughout the entire range of movement. Your legs act like an elevator that lowers your stable upper body into a deep squat all the way toward the floor, low enough that you can reach under the bag of dogfood without disturbing your neutral spine. The moment you begin to lift the bag, you are adding fifty pounds of load to your position. Without generating force from your core and creating stability, your spine will cave in, buckle, or lean to one side in an attempt to manage the load, increasing the forces to your trunk and all the peripheral joints of your body and setting you up for injury due to inadequate core pre-activation.

By recognizing the inherent differences between the sexes, using breath training and trunk exercises to work with (and not against) those differences, educating young girls and boys from an early age about optimal core development and cultivation of body awareness, we can begin to reduce the injury rate gap between men and women and work toward fewer injuries for all.

Seeds for Thought

- Were you surprised to learn about the differences in injury rates between men and women?

- How would you describe your normal way of breathing? Is it deep and from your abdomen, or shallow and from your chest? How do you think this impacts your overall health and performance?

- If you normally breathe from your chest, how did it feel to try deeper breathing?

- Were you able to feel your core muscles activating?

- When performing the pre-activation exercise, what did you notice about your ability to control your descent and ascent with the addition of the counterweight?

CHAPTER 5

Mind-Core Connection

"Only with strong mind and body will you be able to cross the ocean of life."
—Swami Vivekananda

My patient, Jessica, sustained a devastating wakeboarding injury that broke and dislocated her knee while she was shredding at twenty-five miles per hour, rupturing all of her knee ligaments and a major artery in her leg. Time was of the essence for her leg and her life as she held on to her dangling bones, muscles, and tendons while she was pulled onto the boat.

Fortunately, Jessica was quickly airlifted from Wyoming to Utah, where she underwent emergency surgery for a popliteal artery bypass graft to save her leg from amputation and salvage what they could of her knee, where she suffered broken bones and tore her cartilage, tendons, and all four ligaments.

Utilizing her strong mind-core connection, she meditated and focused on her breathing all the way to the hospital. Remarkably, she was able to use deep breathing and meditation to disassociate from her pain. She imagined herself in a "warm sand dune, kissed by a warm breeze that was whisking her pain away as crystals of sand that floated into the blue sky and out into the atmosphere, dispersing through the galaxy." Mindful meditation, deep breathing, and connecting with nature helped her exchange her pain with gratitude for being alive.

In the hospital, the doctors advised her to call and inform her parents that she would likely become an amputee, but she had other plans. Now, just months after her injury, Jessica has made a quick recovery and returned to her work as a wildlife guide and naturalist at Grand Teton and Yellowstone National Parks. She is now sneaking up on buffalo and big horned sheep with a fully functional leg, trekking up to twenty miles per day, and climbing to elevations of 14,000 feet with no knee pain and without any surgical repair or reconstruction on her knee.

Jessica's rehabilitation was undoubtedly so successful because of her resilient mindset and strong mind-body-spirit connection. As a twenty-three-year-old woman, she impressed me with stories of her environmental research, her fearless, worldwide adventures, and her study of nature, meditation, and holistic medicine. Jessica empowered her core not only as an avid hiker, rock climber, kayaker, and snowboarder, but also through her optimism, gratitude, intellectual curiosity, and exploration of alternative philosophies for mindfulness and wellness.

Mind-Core Discoveries

"The joy of discovery is certainly the liveliest
that the mind of man can ever feel."
—Claude Bernard

As a student many years ago, I was taught that after reaching adulthood, the brain had just limited potential for plasticity or neurogenesis (the birth of new neurons). Revolutionary new discoveries are reshaping our understanding of the structure and function of the brain itself, as well as how we view human nature, mental health, and our potential for improving our physical, emotional, and spiritual wellness.

When I began studying healthcare in college, I was taught that our bodies are like machines, and our job as medical professionals was to fix problems when the machine breaks. At the time, alternative and complementary health and medicine practices were not considered evidence-based philosophies, but that has since changed, as more research has demonstrated their benefits. It's always been my goal as a physical therapist to find the broken parts and fix them like a computer technician. The connection between your body and brain is like a computer, and your nervous system is like the software and programming—yet the mind is far more than input and output through circuits and processing.

This mechanistic view of our bodies is now getting an overhaul with revolutionary findings of how the brain works. The relationship between the mind and body has been studied by philosophers, physicians, spiritual sages, and scientific thinkers for thousands of years. Evidence from these various disciplines shows the importance of the mind-core connection for wellness and injury prevention. That means learning to use your mind is a critical component in recovering from injuries or illnesses, and for preventing them.

This new knowledge that our thoughts may physically change the morphology and function of our brains has captured the rapt attention of the neuroscience community. The brain remains much more malleable, or plastic, throughout our lifetimes than we originally believed, which means it is constantly forming and reorganizing new connections in response to our experiences and behaviors. These discoveries have led to some of the most revolutionary and important ideas in modern science. The plasticity of the brain, and how our actions and thoughts can physically change the morphology and function of our minds and bodies, has major implications for emotional well-being, neuromuscular learning, movement deficit correction, and injury prevention.

When you train your core, you create engrams (movement software programs in your nervous system) for complex movements. These engrams dictate which muscles will be used, in which order, and to what degree, then encode these neurological blueprints in the brain and peripheral nervous system. These blueprints allow automatic control processes to operate faster than conscious control of the body.

Core stability training not only empowers your body to avoid injuries, but also has a positive effect on psychological factors such as depression, anxiety, and fear of injury, which has been demonstrated even in people older than sixty-five, proving that your brain and body have the potential to grow and improve throughout your entire lifetime. It's never too late to start training your core for better health!

Meditation Unleashes Your Mind Power

"Meditation is a way of nourishing and blossoming the divinity within you."
—Amit Ray

By making meditation a regular practice, you will strengthen and nurture your mind-body connection, while bringing increased focus and balance to your life. Growing scientific evidence supports the benefits of meditation and mindful breathing for psychological and physical wellness. Recent studies have shown that such mindful activities can reduce stress and anxiety, while improving sleep, self-esteem, focus, memory, problem-solving, and learning. Meditation can also help you manage mood and sleep disorders, as well as post-traumatic stress disorder (PTSD), while also improving your emotional outlook, happiness, self-compassion, ability to adapt to change, and overall quality of life.

In addition to these psychological and cognitive effects, recent evidence also supports physical benefits, most notably pain reduction, improved healing, and reduced inflammation, heart rate, and respiratory rate. Some of the most intriguing recent research has found that mindful meditation may actually affect the gray matter of your brain (the regions involved in muscle control and sensory perception).

When you practice meditation, your breathing rate slows down, which promotes deep breathing that activates the inner core musculature. As you relax your body, you relearn how to breathe properly, turning off the chest breathing muscles you shouldn't be using (the ones that cause tension and headaches), and turning on your core deep breathing muscles. Full engagement of the core muscles increases efficiency of your lungs and makes your breathing more effective, which is important for mind-body health and core stabilization.

You can boost your mood and strengthen your core by using three complementary, scientifically-based meditation strategies to achieve mindful breathing and awareness of your core for empowerment: Focused Attention Meditation, Open Monitoring Meditation, and Transcendental Meditation. These strategies will help your mind and body stay resilient to keep you on an even keel and help you weather the storms of life. In this chapter, you will learn the general concepts of these strategies so you can start practicing them. Strength and stability of your mind are essential for strength and stability of your core!

Core-Empowering Meditations

Focused Attention Meditation (FAM)

"There's only here. There's only now."
—Van Morrison

To practice Focused Attention Meditation, direct your attention to a specific experience or feeling, beginning with a full-body scan from head to toe, without allowing your mind to wander. Mentally examine your body for areas where you may be holding tension, then consciously release or soften these areas individually to a complete state of relaxation. This meditation approach is an excellent starting point to help the novice meditator turn off their multi-tasking mind and stay in the present moment.

Learning to sense the activation and release of your muscles provides body-to-mind feedback and is an essential skill for establishing mind-to-core control. In fact, recent studies show that FAM promotes increased brain power and coherence, or connectivity within the brain.

The FAM strategy establishes the mind-core foundation of core stability by regulating your nervous system, training your proprioception, and deepening your understanding of your own core alignment, breathing mechanics, and core muscle activation.

Open Monitoring (or Zen) Meditation (OMM)

"The secret of health for both mind and body is not to mourn the past, not to worry about the future, but to live in the present moment."
—Buddha

Open Monitoring Meditation, also known as "open attention" or "soft focus" meditation, requires you to simply observe your mind and body without reacting, and without judgement. Begin OMM by practicing awareness of your thoughts and experiences from moment to moment, through your natural stream of consciousness. This means taking the time to notice your thoughts, emotions, and senses. Allow this sensory information to arise and simply float away as new sensations float in.

Your goal is to keep your mind in the monitoring state so you can achieve awareness of breath, posture, and core function in the present moment. This is when the insight you need for core empowerment is best developed. To observe your core, distance yourself so that you are witnessing, rather than thinking, interacting, or controlling. Let go of the past and the future without attempting to control your thoughts.

Research shows that OMM is particularly effective at calming the mind and nervous system, which improves brain activity associated with heightened attention, focus, and muscle memory. Activating the core musculature and developing core awareness requires all of these components.

Transcendental Meditation (TM)

"Your body is not who you are. The mind and spirit transcend the body."
—Christopher Reeve

To begin Transcendental Meditation for mind-core integration, think an empowering thought. Begin with a simple word or phrase that you repeat in your mind over and over in a relaxed way. For example, you could repeat the word "relax" in your mind as you practice TM. Your brain and body will believe what you tell it. Let go of negative thoughts such as "I am not good enough" and embrace positive affirmations, such as "I have unlimited potential." The goal of TM is to develop a higher state of consciousness, a deeper understanding of spiritual meaning, and a connection with a higher power, whether through prayer or by connecting with the energy around you.

Recent studies show this form of meditation increases blood flow to attention areas of the brain and decreases blood flow to the arousal areas of the brain. Thus, TM reduces distraction, stress, anxiety, and blood pressure, while improving clarity, focus, cognition, creativity, energy, proprioception, and balance. This mind-core practice allows your conscious mind to take a backseat so your deep unconscious mind can surface, which facilitates transcendence to new levels of core awareness and multiplies your potential for core empowerment.

Be patient as you practice meditation and find your own path to connecting with yourself. There is no right or wrong way to meditate, as long as your intention is clear and your mind is free of distractions. Regardless of how packed your schedule is, it's important to set aside time for meditation in order to empower your body and mind, and center your core like the stable eye of a hurricane.

Mind-Core Empowering Strategies

Mindful Breathing Exercise

"Breath is the bridge which connects life to consciousness, which unites your body to your thoughts. Whenever your mind becomes scattered, use your breath as the means to take hold of your mind again."
—Thich Nhat Hanh

Siddhartha Gautama, also known as Buddha, recognized this important connection between the mind and body during the sixth century BC, yet scientists are only just beginning to understand the incredible benefits of meditation and mindfulness training.

Mindfulness is a mental state of focused awareness in the present moment, beginning with close attention to your breath and calm acceptance of your thoughts, feelings, and bodily sensations. Mindful core breathing is the practice of meditating and tuning in completely to the experience of deep diaphragmatic breathing and core activation. It is also an essential empowering component of the Core BASE Guide.

You can use this focus on breathing and core activation to explore what is unknown about your mind and body, so you can bring into consciousness what has been unconscious. This is a learning process, and the information you learn while meditating and practicing mindfulness can help you improve your mental and physical health and performance in just about every area of life. Your breath is a bridge between your mind and nervous system, because the breath functions both consciously and unconsciously. You can control your breath, yet when you stop trying to control it, your breath continues without any prompting.

The art of breath training for wellness has been practiced for thousands of years in Eastern cultures and has become increasingly popular in the West due to growing research of holistic wellness. By practicing mindful breathing exercises at least five minutes each day, you will learn to focus your attention on your own breathing, clear your restless mind, and slip into stillness.

To get started, choose a quiet and comfortable place. Close your eyes and relax all the muscles of your body as you journey to inner peace. Feel the sense of lightness in your trunk as you inhale and exhale.

If you feel stressed, it helps to start with an exaggerated breath. Take a deep, long inhale through your nose, and a slightly longer exhale out your nose. Breathing through your nose, as opposed to your mouth, is the best way for you to breathe, because your nose filters the air of allergens and foreign bodies. Breath that has passed through your nasal passage is warmed and moistened, which inhibits bacteria and viruses, promoting optimal oxygenation for every cell in your body.

Next, simply turn your awareness to your body. Observe your natural breath without trying to regulate it. By paying attention to all of your physical sensations, you can take your mind off the barrage of wandering thoughts that might normally keep you tense throughout the day. Focus all of your attention on your body. Mentally scan your body to see if you have any areas of pain or tension and breathe into these areas to release tension and relax. Move your conscious awareness throughout every part of your body, focusing on one particular muscle group at a time.

If your mind begins to wander, simply imagine the thoughts floating away with your exhalations, and gently bring your awareness back to the rise and fall of your chest and belly. Practicing mindful breathing will make it easier to focus attention on your breath as your anchor in everyday life, which can help you cope with stress and develop your mind-core connection.

Mindful Meditation During All Activities

"If you have time to breathe, you have time to meditate."
—Ajahn Amaro

Breath work is a critical component of meditation. Focusing attention on your breath naturally takes attention away from your thoughts and stressors. Mindful meditation can be practiced anytime, anywhere. No matter what you are doing, you can mentally tune in to your breathing patterns and observe the flow of your breath without any judgment or criticism. There is no wrong way to meditate, just like there is no wrong way to feel sunshine on your face. Meditation can be as simple as admiring the colors of a sunset, savoring the smell of lavender, or feeling a sea breeze.

Tune in to your core with mindful meditation to center yourself and brighten your day in the morning, to decompress at bedtime for restful sleep, or to relax while performing your usual activities during the day. During intense exercise, your breath is naturally going to be deeper to meet the demands of your cardiovascular system. Regardless of the intensity level, tuning in to your breathing promotes a meditative mindset. Exercise mindfully and train your mind like you would any other muscle in your body. Research shows that what you focus on while exercising can actually improve your brain's ability to signal muscle activity and change your muscles' morphology (making them bigger and stronger).

Meditating while walking is an excellent way to start practicing, because you can learn what it feels like to be mindful while performing a familiar activity. (It can be more difficult to meditate during more complex activities that are new to you.) Pay attention to your breathing and any sensations you feel in your body as your feet hit the ground. Notice the way your core moves, and the way your arms coordinate with your trunk and your lower body to propel you forward. Focus on releasing tension, particularly in your shoulders and neck, where tension typically accumulates. Enjoy the experience of movement and soak in the beauty around you.

If you are not fortunate enough to be surrounded by natural beauty, try utilizing guided imagery, a form of mindful meditation that uses the mind to focus on positive images and thoughts to promote well-being and relaxation. Guided imagery uses visualization to enhance awareness of the mind-body connection to improve balance, strength, and cardiovascular health, ease performance anxiety, and help you excel in sports. Use your imagination to transport your mind to a place that brings you peace and joy, focusing on what all of your senses are soaking in: the sound of chirping birds, turquoise ocean waves, or the fragrance of honeysuckle blooms.

Since the body and the mind are interconnected, you can use guided imagery to actually experience what you are imagining while connecting to your breath and your core. Transfer these skills while tuning in to your breath during fun core activities that target and empower your core, such as Pilates, yoga, martial arts, singing, dancing, laughing, sports, adventures in nature, or the Core BASE exercises in Part 2 of this book.

Reframing Negative Thoughts into Positive Thoughts

"Keep your face in the sunshine and you will not see a shadow."
—Helen Keller

Negative thoughts can hinder your ability to function at your optimal level, and they're counterproductive to your aspirations. In fact, studies show that fear and lack of confidence are strong predictors of injury. Don't let self-doubt or senseless worries keep you and your core down! A useful strategy to turn blue thoughts into true thoughts is to recognize the negative thoughts and write them down, like when you think "I'm not strong enough, fast enough, or skilled enough." These thoughts from your harsh inner critic focus negative energy on your weaknesses and perceived flaws. Negative self-talk results in low self-esteem, a lack of confidence, and unhappiness.

Ask yourself how you can transform these thoughts into positive affirmations by flipping them 180 degrees and focusing on your goals and your progress toward these goals, no matter how small. Instead of striving for achievement and recognition because you don't feel like you're good enough yet, pursue your goals because they are good for you and because they will help you stretch, grow, and empower yourself.

Positive thinking is a practice. Like working out, it takes effort but becomes habitual over time. Use positive self-talk to reframe the destructive habits of comparing yourself to others, or worrying too much about what others think of you. We are all surrounded by positivity and negativity in our lives, but you get to choose how to respond and what to focus on. Concentrating on your achievements, setting realistic goals, and having patience with your progress are all characteristics of a healthy growth mindset.

Exercising your brain onto a positive track creates positive neuropathways, just like exercising your muscles. Instead of succumbing and being pushed around by the unpredictable waves of life, take responsibility and control of your thoughts and attitude. When you substitute negative beliefs with positive ones, you will begin to notice positive results.

Practicing Gratitude

"Gratitude opens the door to the power, the wisdom, the creativity of
the universe. You open the door through gratitude."
—Deepak Chopra

Gratitude is the quality, long valued by ancient moral philosophies,
of being thankful, appreciative, and ready to return kindness. You can
practice gratitude by pausing to acknowledge and appreciate all the
good in yourself and your surroundings. Thanking yourself, thanking
others, and thanking the universe will help you achieve a stable mind
and core.

Many studies over the past decade have shown that being grateful
will improve both your mental and physical health. Being thankful has
significant correlations with the central nervous system that we are
just beginning to discover, including greater areas of grey matter in the
brain and the release of dopamine and serotonin neurotransmitters,
which are your "feel good" chemical messengers.

Gratefulness can benefit your body through improved immune
and cardiovascular health, better sleep, more happiness, increased
productivity, deeper emotional awareness, and enhanced participation
and adherence to exercise and healthy lifestyle choices.

Practicing gratitude also decreases negative emotions such as envy,
anger, anxiety, and depression. So take a deep, mindful breath and
remind yourself how grateful you are for everything in your life! Your
spirit will thank you with improved self-esteem, self-satisfaction, and
vitality, and the universe will reward you with good karma and health.

Mindful Meditation to Relieve Pain

"The purpose of meditation is to awaken in us the sky-like nature
of mind, and to introduce us to that which we really are, our
unchanging pure awareness."
—Sogyal Rinpoche

Each year, millions of people suffer from pain due to injuries and
disease. Chronic pain affects over 100 million Americans, with $635
billion lost annually in medical expenses or work productivity. Living

with pain also affects quality of life by creating emotional strain, with feelings of frustration, depression, anger, and despair. Until recently, medication was the most widespread pain management option, but due to the opioid epidemic, the medical profession is shifting away from drugs as the answer for pain.

Unlike drugs that create unpleasant side effects, disturbed mental balance, and the threat of addiction, meditation is becoming a popular method for naturally and effectively managing pain. New evidence, revealed in MRI (magnetic resonance imaging) testing of the brain, shows a significant decrease in pain perception in people who meditate. Mindful meditation actually changes the way the brain perceives pain to make it more tolerable. The ability to cope with pain improves, and in turn, alleviates the mental and emotional strain associated with pain, without any risks or negative side effects.

Pain also causes changes in muscle activation (delayed and inadequate activation, and decreased endurance), which further compromises stabilization and control of your spine. Re-educating the core muscles to work synergistically with diaphragmatic breathing reduces back pain and enhances stability of your spine and your entire body's chain of segments. Keeping your mind in tune with your breath to awaken your core helps break this vicious cycle of pain, compromised core stability, and injury.

We will all experience pain at some point in our lives. Back pain, for instance, is the most common musculoskeletal ailment in the United States, but it can be mitigated with core training. Many studies have shown that training your core muscles to create a "natural corset" of support for your spine helps alleviate back pain. This muscular corset will better equip your body to handle physical stress from your everyday life, your workouts, and sports. Without a strong and stable core, your body will rely more on the passive structures of your spine (ligaments, bones, and joints), which puts more stress on your spinal discs and increases your likelihood of sustaining injuries and pain.

Training your mind-core connection with core stability exercises will improve your neuromuscular control, strength, and endurance of your trunk, which is necessary for dynamic stability and protection of all parts of your body. Ultimately, your mind and core are one, and training them together will greatly impact what your body can achieve!

Seeds for Thought

- Did you try the three different types of meditation? How did they feel?

- What, if anything, did you find challenging about these activities?

- Do you recognize negative thoughts and practice substituting with positive affirmations and gratitude?

- If this was your first time, how was the experience?

- How did practicing mindfulness in one of your daily activities change the way you experienced that activity, and how did you feel afterward?

CHAPTER 6

Heart-Core Connection

"In hardness, tension, general strength, and resistance to injury, the fibers of the heart far surpass all others, for no other instrument performs such continuous, hard work as the heart."
—Aristotle

Aristotle and other ancient philosophers, including Greeks, Egyptians, Arabs, and Indians, believed that the heart controls sensation, thoughts, and movement, and is the organ most closely related to the soul. Although this cardio-centric philosophy of human functioning has fallen from modern medicine (which has since demonstrated that the brain plays the dominant role in controlling the body), there is no question that the heart and the core have an intricately linked anatomical and functional relationship.

The fibrous pericardium, or the connective tissue sac that encapsulates the heart, is continuous with the roof of the core (the diaphragm muscle) and the abdominal connective tissue down to the pelvic floor. The diaphragm is also connected to the heart by a tendon, a thick cord that attaches to the pericardium. When the diaphragm muscle contracts, this tendon tugs downward on the pericardium with a tight hug around the heart. With each breath, your heart rides up and down with the momentum of the diaphragm, as blood flow and neural information is relayed between the thoracic cavity of the chest and the abdominal cavity of the core.

This synchronous action of the core that you experience during cardiovascular exercise reduces the risk of heart disease, obesity, stroke, diabetes, high blood pressure, cancer, and complications related to pregnancy. Other studies show that cardio improves cognitive function, including your memory and reasoning skills, while slowing the decline of brain function that comes with aging and dementia. Other studies show that getting your heart pumping promotes better bone health and balance, lowering your risk of injury from falls.

The physical link of the nervous system between your heart and your core affects you in profound ways. The nerves in your diaphragm affect your heart rate and blood pressure, and reduce stress in the body by lowering stress hormones. These stress hormones have a lot of negative effects on your mind-body-spirit and have even been shown to cause excess belly fat.

Cardiovascular exercise can lift your mood, decrease anxiety, and fight depression. If you are feeling down, exercise may seem to be the farthest thing from your mind, but studies show that exercise releases "feel good" chemicals in your brain to pull you out of the dumps, distract you in a positive way from a cycle of negative thoughts and emotions that are harmful to your health, and trigger a feeling of elation and euphoria. Work your core and your heart together to help you think, feel, and sleep better for a better quality of life and sense of overall well-being!

Injury and Heart Health

"Injuries are our best teachers."
—Scott Jurek

Recently, a group of investigators at Harvard found that athletes who suffered from ACL tears had double the chance of experiencing a heart attack later in life. This connection between the heart and a ligament in your knee has raised some eyebrows among clinicians and researchers. The investigators even accounted for other possible contributing factors to heart problems, such as smoking, obesity, age, and race. One possible explanation for this intriguing new revelation is that ACL tears create chronic inflammation throughout the body, which may possibly contribute to blockage in one or more of the vessels that supply blood to the heart.

Another hypothesis is that immobilization and loss of activity following trauma has a detrimental effect on your heart. This is not surprising to me, as over the years I have seen many patients whose shattered dreams, resulting from these and other devastating injuries, have left them in hopeless despair. Many fall from the extreme of peak fitness to the extreme of a completely sedentary lifestyle. Even those who may not be elite athletes struggle with long term repercussions as a result of their injuries, which impact their outlook and quality of life. Inactivity is a major health concern in modern society, especially in urban areas, contributing to cardiovascular problems and premature mortality. Heart disease is the leading cause of death in the world, and living a sedentary lifestyle is one of the biggest contributors to this massive health issue.

Being physically active is critical for a healthy heart. It is the most effective tool for strengthening your heart muscle, minimizing damage to your blood vessels that can cause heart attacks and strokes, and keeping your weight under control. The American Heart Association recommends two and a half hours of heart-pumping exercise (such as running, spinning, elliptical, swimming, or power walking) per week, yet only 20 percent of adults and children get enough exercise to truly nourish their hearts. Children should get one hour of moderate exercise per day, which can include sports, gym class, or just running around playing tag. These guidelines are based on current scientific evidence that supports the importance of moderate physical activity for heart and overall health.

Tuning in to Your Heart

"Everything in moderation."
—Ancient Greek Proverb

Hopefully by now I've convinced you of the importance of getting your heart pumping, both for your overall health and the strength of your core, so you can prevent more injuries. But how do you gauge the intensity to make sure you're exercising enough, without overdoing it? For any aerobic activity, exercise intensity correlates with how hard the activity feels to you, or your perceived exertion. If you think you're working hard, your heart rate is probably higher than usual. This may be different from what someone else feels doing the same exercise. For example, what seems to you like a grueling hike can feel like an easy stroll to someone who's more fit.

Tune in to your heart and your body's response to exercise by looking out for some tell-tale signs that can help you judge your exercise intensity. Moderate activity feels somewhat difficult and causes your breath to quicken, but you should still be able to carry on a conversation. Generally, you'll break a light sweat after about five to ten minutes of such activity. Intense or vigorous activity feels more challenging. Some clues that your exercise intensity is at a vigorous level include rapid, gasping breath and sweating soon after initiating activity (within five minutes). It's important to build intensity slowly and steadily. Don't push yourself too hard, as this may actually be detrimental to your heart and your health.

You might think that training at high intensity is the best way to get stronger, faster, or improve your performance in sports, but you'd be wrong. Elite endurance athletes spend most of their time training in the green zone (a moderate activity level where they can still carry on a full conversation the entire time). Many athletes and weekend warriors suffer injuries by pushing themselves too hard and too fast. Not only is this a dangerous strategy, but it's not optimal for increasing athletic performance either.

Let's Get Heart Smart!

To more objectively assess your exercise intensity, you can monitor your heart rate. Your heart rate, or pulse, is the number of times your heart beats per minute during exercise. Normal heart rate varies from person to person. The higher your heart rate during physical activity, the higher the intensity. To use this method of assessing your workouts, you must first learn how to check your pulse. Monitor your pulse a few times per week and at different times of the day to get a real-time snapshot of how your heart is functioning.

Checking Your Pulse

"At the heart of each of us, whatever our imperfections, there exists a silent pulse of perfect rhythm, which is absolutely individual and unique, and yet which connects us to everything else."
—George Leonard

To check your pulse over your carotid artery, place your index and middle fingers on your neck, to the side of your throat. Do not use your thumb, because it has its own artery and pulse that you may feel, which can make it more difficult to count accurately. You can also check your pulse by placing two fingers lightly on your radial artery, located on the thumb side of your wrist, for thirty seconds. Multiply this number by two to calculate your heart beats per minute. Even if you're not an athlete, knowledge about your heart rate can help you monitor your fitness level and may help you identify developing health issues.

Your resting heart rate is the number of times your heart beats when you are relaxed. The American Heart Association recommends checking your resting heart rate first thing in the morning, before you get out of bed. At this time, your heart is pumping out the lowest amount of blood you need to function, because you're not exercising. If you're sitting or lying down and you're calm, your heart rate is normally between 60 and 100 beats per minute. However, a heart rate lower than 60 doesn't necessarily signal a medical problem. Keep in mind that the number can be influenced by many factors, such as hormones, and medications like antidepressants or blood pressure drugs.

A lower heart rate is also common in people who get a lot of physical activity, or who are very athletic. Active people often have a lower resting heart rate (as low as 40) because their heart muscle is in better condition and doesn't need to work as hard to maintain a steady beat. If you are not on medication or are not very fit, a low pulse or an unexplained fast heart rate, especially if you feel weak or dizzy, is reason to tell your doctor. Your pulse is one tool that can offer a picture of your overall health.

Calculating Your Maximum Heart Rate

"Life isn't measured in minutes, but in heartbeats."
—Joan Lowery Nixon

The next step is to calculate an estimate of your maximum heart rate. This is the limit of what your heart can handle, or the highest your pulse can get. You can roughly predict your maximum heart rate by subtracting your age from 220. For example, if you're 35 years old, subtract 35 from 220 to get a maximum heart rate of 185 beats per minute. This is the maximum number of times your heart beats per minute. Keep in mind that this is an estimate. Your true maximum heart rate could be as many as 15 beats higher or lower than your calculation from this formula.

Once you know your maximum heart rate, you can calculate your desired target heart rate zone, or the level at which your heart is being conditioned, but not strained. When you are exercising, this is the range where you gain the most benefits with the least amount of risk. It is the heart rate you should aim for when exercising.

The American Heart Association recommends a target heart rate of about 50 to 70 percent of your maximum heart rate for moderate cardio, and 70 to 85 percent of your maximum heart rate for vigorous exercise intensity. It is not recommended to exercise above 85 percent of your maximum heart rate, as doing so can increase your health risk and does not add any extra benefit. If you're not in great shape yet, stay in the lower end of your target heart rate zone.

Progressively build the intensity of exercise. If you're healthy and want a good heart workout, aim for the higher end of the moderate zone. If you want a more specific range, consider discussing your target heart rate zone with a doctor, physical therapist, or exercise physiologist. You may also need to use a lower target heart rate zone because of your medications or medical conditions.

Interval training involves moderate exercise, but with 30- to 60-second bouts of higher intensity exercise spread throughout your workout. This is great for burning fat to promote weight loss, and is well tolerated even in those with mild heart disease and diabetes. Before starting a vigorous exercise program, you may want to talk with your doctor. He or she may suggest that you have certain tests done first. This is true especially for people who have health problems, and for men over age forty-five or women over age fifty-five.

Use Your "Wandering" Nerve to Find Heart Health

"To be calm is the highest achievement of the self."
—Yogi Bhajan

Heart health is not just about elevating your heart rate with exercise; slowing your heart rate is equally important. The vagus nerve, the key player in regulating heart rate, is the longest nerve in your body and it connects your brain to many other important organs. (There are actually two, but they're commonly referred to in the singular form.) The word "vagus" means "wanderer" in Latin, which accurately represents how the nerve travels through many organs from your head to your chest and your abdomen, branching out to the gut (your intestines and stomach), heart, and lungs. This critical nerve is also a key part of your parasympathetic nervous system. The wandering nerve is associated with a multitude of important functions, including swallowing, tasting, breathing, digesting, and maintaining your heart rate, all of which can have a huge impact on your mind-body-spirit health. Vagal activation sends a signal to your brain that all is well to relax you and reassure your heart and mind.

The "tone" of your vagus nerve represents the activity and functionality of this important nerve. Increasing your vagal tone activates the parasympathetic nervous system, and having higher vagal tone means that your body can return to a relaxed state more quickly after stress. There is a positive feedback loop between high vagal tone, positive emotions, and good physical health. In other words, the more you increase your vagal tone, the more your physical and mental health will improve, and vice versa. Vagal tone lowers the resting heart rate, regulates mood, provides relief from headaches, improves immune function, provides mental clarity, and creates an overall feeling of peace and happiness.

A poorly functioning vagus nerve, or one with reduced vagal tone, is associated with the release of stress hormones that contribute to chronic inflammation, which leads to heart disease and many other health repercussions. A healthy vagus nerve helps to keep stress and inflammation levels low, and can reduce your risk of developing heart disease. Studies have even shown that vagal tone is passed on from mother to child. Mothers who are depressed, anxious, and angry during their pregnancy have lower vagal activity. Once they give birth to their child, the newborn also has low vagal activity and low dopamine and serotonin levels, which are chemical messengers in your nervous system that affect mood, digestion, and sleep.

Your vagal tone can be measured by your heart rate, breathing rate, and what's called heart rate variability, or the variance in time between beats of your heart. Your heart rate variability is a major indicator of the intrinsic nervous system of the heart. The more variable your heart rate, the more resilient and healthier your heart is. When your heart rate variability is high, your vagal tone is also high. The gold standard for measuring heart rate variability is to analyze a long strip of an electrocardiogram, a test your doctor can do by attaching wires to your chest and monitoring the electrical activity of your heart. You can also buy a chest strap monitor and use an online app to analyze the data and get in tune with your heartbeat, the fundamental rhythm of life.

Strategies to Stimulate Your Vagus Nerve

"Make your heart like a lake, with a calm, still surface, and great depths of kindness."
—Lao Tzu

Deep and slow mindful breathing and meditation are effective ways of increasing your vagal tone and lowering your heart rate, reducing anxiety, and helping you reach a state of relaxation. You can try some other simple, scientifically-based methods as described below to stimulate your vagus nerve. This will allow you to respond more effectively to the physical, emotional, and physiological stressors of life. Now take a breath and try these simple tips for chilling out!

Chill

"If you tiptoe into cold water, you're missing out on the rush of plunging in headfirst."
—Simone Elkeles

The slang expression "chill out," meaning to "relax" or "calm down," is believed to have originated in the 1970s, popularized by the Sugar Hill Gang song "Rapper's Delight." Who could have foreseen that this catchy expression coined by funky rappers would someday be backed by modern science, which has demonstrated that cold exposure prompts the vagus nerve to actually "chill" you out? This vagal stimulation lowers the sympathetic "fight or flight" response, increases parasympathetic activity, lowers your heart rate, and induces relaxation. Try finishing your next shower or bath by rinsing for thirty seconds with chilly water. If you are pressed for time or are having a stressful day away from home, try splashing your face with cold water in a sink to chill.

"Bee" Calm

"Let it be."
—The Beatles

Your vagus nerve is connected to your vocal cords and the muscles at the back of your throat. When you buzz like a bee, hum, chant, or gargle, you activate these structures and stimulate your vagus nerve. Try "buzzing" or humming like a bee while exhaling as slowly as possible through your nose. Take long, deep inhalations, and even slower exhalations. Humming, or lengthened exhalation through the nose while making an "mmm" sound, generates positive vibrations—literally! Research indicates that buzzing, humming, or chanting the word "om" stimulates the vagus nerve and helps put the body in a state of relaxation, boosting mind power and providing mental clarity.

Give Your Vagus Some Love

"To touch can be to give life."
—Michelangelo

The benefits of massage are well documented, and include reduced stress and muscle tension. New studies demonstrate that massaging specific areas of your body stimulates the vagus nerve and increases vagal tone. Stimulating the vagus nerve is like pressing a button that tells your body it's time to relax and de-stress, which leads to long-term improvements in mood and heart health. Increasing vagal tone will allow you to overcome anxiety and depression, and better manage these conditions when they arise. A poorly functioning vagus nerve is linked to poor health and chronic disease, whereas a well-functioning and healthy vagus nerve is essential for your heart and overall mind-body-spirit health. Massages have been shown to increase vagal modulation and heart rate variability while decreasing the sympathetic response.

Sex-Related Differences in Heart Health

"Your feet will take you where your heart is."
—Irish and Ukrainian Proverb

The landscape of women's participation in sports has dramatically changed over the past century. When I ran the Boston marathon in an equal sea of female and male runners, it was hard to believe that fewer than fifty years prior, women were not even allowed to qualify and had to sneak into the race. Female sports participation has skyrocketed, yet women account for only 3 percent of study participants in medical research, creating a huge knowledge gap. Exercise studies have traditionally been performed on predominantly male subjects, defining norms in terms of a typical 155-pound man and working under the misguided assumption that female and male bodies are essentially the same.

For years, female athletes had to rely on training protocols that were based on this male-focused research. The lack of female inclusion in studies was mostly due to the facts that men were the primary investigators, more male athletes were available as subjects, and more funding was available for male sports. This imbalance of important information inspired me to do my own research and improve our understanding of female exercise and injury prevalence. There is now growing recognition that women experience training, injury, and recovery differently than men, and that women would benefit from sex-specific research and guidelines.

Important sex-related differences in the physiological response to exercise are finally being recognized. Female hormonal fluctuation affects the way women regulate their body temperatures, how they metabolize nutrients, and how they maintain hydration, which influences performance and recovery. When women start their periods, hormone levels drop. During this time, women can easily metabolize carbohydrates and experience less fatigue. This is a great time for women to get their hearts pumping to witness significant improvements in their training.

As hormone levels increase, cramps, bloating, digestive issues, and elevated body temperature make exercise more challenging. During this time of high hormonal levels, it's more difficult for a woman's body to metabolize carbohydrates and repair muscles. It is important for women to get in tune with their cycles and recognize how those cycles affect their bodies so they can adjust their training accordingly. If you are hoping to trim your figure as well as nourish your heart, opt for interval training instead of a long, steady exercise to burn any excess fat you're trying to get rid of.

Long, steady cardio works better for men, as men burn stubborn belly and lower body fat more easily than women. Women's bodies are designed to preserve the lower body fat, even when exercising for long, steady intensities, which is why we see so many pear-shaped runners. Many women who run marathons have bodies that are still trying to preserve the excess weight in their lower bodies.

Studies show that it is healthier to have a big rear end and thighs than a huge stomach, yet many women feel self-conscious about their pear shape. Women can boost their calorie burn and weight loss benefits by including intervals. Interval training is unrivaled when it comes to preventing heart disease, losing weight, and improving overall fitness. No matter what form of aerobic exercise you choose, mix in thirty to sixty seconds of higher-intensity activity every few minutes, in the upper limit of your target heart rate zone. This will get your heart pumping faster, clear fat and sugar from your blood, and transform your pear into an hourglass.

Men still have physiological advantages when it comes to strength and power. However, recent evidence shows that women do have the edge in extreme endurance activities, like ultra-marathons, especially exercise that takes place in a warm environment. Thanks to our tough hunter-gatherer female ancestors, who carried their children for thousands of miles, women have inherited the ability to conserve muscle energy and release heat more efficiently than men. This adaptation is thought to be due to the greater muscle mass in men. It is believed that women have evolved to maintain their body temperatures by reducing blood flow to the skin.

Regardless of who has the advantage, men and women have many physiological similarities, and both have the ability to increase their strength, power, and endurance through a commitment to cardiovascular exercise for mind, body, and spiritual wellness. You can't beat a healthy heart!

Seeds for Thought

- When you checked your pulse, was your resting heart rate within the target range?

- How do you usually feel after cardiovascular exercise?

- Do your workouts usually consist of high-intensity exercises, or more moderate cardio activities?

- Are you able to carry on a conversation while you are exercising?

- What types of strategies can you incorporate into your daily life to increase vagal tone for mind-body-spirit health?

CHAPTER 7

Core Holistic Nourishment

"The organs are the horses, the mind is the rein, the intellect is the
charioteer, the soul is the rider, and the body is the chariot."
—Swami Vivekananda

Your well-being comes not just from your physical health, but also
from your mental, emotional, and spiritual health. All these aspects
of your nature are interdependent, like getting a headache when you
feel anxious, being depressed when you don't exercise, eating too much
because you're nervous, or experiencing that awesome peaceful feeling
when you pray, go to the spa, or practice yoga. That is your mind, body,
and spirit all working together to make you feel whole and happy. A
tri-directional relationship exists between your body, mind, and soul.
How you feel, your posture, your facial expressions, the energy you exude,
and how you absorb the energy of others and the universe around you all
influence your emotions and outlook. For example, simply assuming a
body posture of power influences hormone levels, increases performance,
and can help you to cope better during stressful situations.

The main concept behind mind-body-spirit health is that we are
all more than just our bodies. We are also our thoughts, our emotions,
and our spirituality, which combine to give us identity, determine our
health, and make us who we are, and who our children will be. You must
nourish your body, mind, and spirit to flourish!

Nourish Your Genes

"The apple does not fall far from the tree."
—Ralph Waldo Emerson

I will never forget the amazement in my students' eyes when they
would dissect gorillas, monkeys, and humans in the Comparative
Primate Anatomy Laboratory, and realize that these bodies were all
anatomically similar in terms of bones, muscles, tendons, ligaments,

organs, and blood vessels. We share 99 percent of our genes with our closest relatives, the apes, and yet most of us behave much differently than chimps or bonobos.

Recent scientific advancements have shed some light on what separates us from these primates. It is not just the genes we have, but also how they're regulated that makes us who we are. Similar genes can give rise to different organisms when the genes are activated differently. The future of an apple seed is influenced not only by the tree it came from (and the trees that produced the seeds of the trees before it), but also by its environment in terms of sun, water, nutrients, wind, temperature, and many other factors.

Anyone who has a green thumb will attest that nurturing plants with love helps them to thrive. "Nature" and "nurture" work together to shape all living things, including the people we are. That's because genes are just a blueprint that allow our cells to create proteins, but our bodies have to constantly decide which genes to activate and which genes not to activate, and it's all those little choices our cells make that determine our genetic expression.

Positive environments, experiences, and emotions (such as happiness, creativity, empathy, and love) all influence the choices our cells make and improve our genetic expression. Growing evidence suggests that we can rewrite our genetic destiny that has been passed down to us. New evidence is indicating that, while our genes are our predisposition, they are not necessarily our destiny, nor the destiny of our children. We can actually change the way our DNA is expressed in our bodies to better fight lifestyle-related diseases, including obesity, diabetes, cancer, heart disease, and many others that we are just beginning to discover. Our bodies have a natural wisdom with intrinsic knowledge of how to grow, heal, balance, and regenerate.

Recent neuroscientific research shows that having positive mindset and disposition (focusing attention toward the good in life) promotes new brain growth through the reinforcement and generation of new synapses, or connections. Training your mind to see something good in every situation improves your brain's ability to function, but also strengthens your physical and emotional capacity, making you healthier in body and spirit. A plethora of recent scientific evidence shows that meditating, practicing gratitude, and reframing negative thoughts into positive affirmations can physically transform the brain and improve your health. So if you think of your body as an operating system, it is important to not only upgrade the hardware of your physical body, but also the software of your mindset.

Self-Love Transforms Your Mind-Body-Spirit

"Self-care is how you take your power back."
—Lalah Delia

Recent studies have shown that your beliefs, experiences, and life choices have been influenced by your parents and their ancestors, and will affect your children, their children, and generations to come, proving that your experiences matter beyond each fleeting moment. How you live your life, how your body functions, and how you nurture your mind and body today can change how your DNA functions tomorrow and for years to come.

We inherit both our strengths and our vulnerabilities from our DNA and from environmental factors, such as inherited family lifestyle choices and emotional patterns passed down to us across multiple generations. Epigenetics, the promising new study of gene expression, shows that how we take care of our mind-body-spirit will influence the expression of genes and will have a profound effect on the future of all humankind. In fact, epigenetics means "on top" or "above" our genes in Latin. Epigenetic changes alter the physical structure of our DNA by turning some genes "on" and some genes "off."

You have the power to make enduring changes in the tissues of your brain that affect your future functioning and wellness. If you feel like self-care is selfish, just trust in these science-backed reasons for being kind to yourself, practicing self-love, adopting a positive perspective, cultivating wholesome experiences, and using the core empowering strategies of the Core BASE Guide. This program will help you to reduce your risk of injury, promote your health, and truly flourish in your life while improving the DNA you'll pass on to future generations.

We have evolved over millions of years with these inherent abilities, yet this evolution is influenced by our mindsets and the lifestyle choices we make, including what we think, eat, or drink; how we manage stress; and how much we exercise, sleep, or take time for self-care. We have the ability to change our own genetic blueprints for ourselves and for our children. See if you can recognize any behaviors or vulnerabilities that you may have inherited. Put a plan in place to deepen your self-awareness and self-regulation of your behaviors, and choose what will nourish and empower the DNA of your family tree. Your body is more than the sum of its parts; it has an energy, or life force, that goes beyond the mere physical nature of your body or your generation.

> "Everything is energy and that's all there is to it."
> —Albert Einstein

We are all filled with energy. For thousands of years, ancient philosophies have associated the force of life energy with the health of our physical, emotional, and spiritual selves. This universal energy is called "Qi" in China, "Ki" in Japan, "Prana" in India, "Mana" in Polynesia, "Ruach" in Hebrew, and "Baraka" in Islam. For thousands of years, all these cultures have believed that this energy is what nourishes and sustains life, while stagnation or imbalance of this energy contributes to disease and injury.

Modern science is also beginning to recognize the value of this energy, thanks to research that was more recently developed by Einstein in his famous energy theories. In his final letter to his daughter, Einstein wrote about the "most powerful force of all that governs all others—the universal force of love, which has limitless power to give force to life and energy to heal the world." Nourish your mind-body-spirit with love by making lifestyle choices that will power your core.

High-Grade Fuel

> "May the nourishment of the earth be yours."
> —John O'Donohue

Fill your tank with high-grade fuel by feeding your body wisely! Muscle strength, endurance, and power are contingent upon adequate core nourishment, and are critical in maintaining healthy posture, spinal stability, and core wellness. Muscle fatigue contributes to instability and injury. Optimal nourishment for core musculature requires a diverse, holistic diet, yet unfortunately, many people rely on processed and manufactured foods that do not meet core nutritional requirements. Each year, over 500,000 Americans die prematurely of poor diet!

Hallmarks of core holistic nutrition include organic, unprocessed, unrefined, and locally grown whole foods. These include fruits, vegetables, whole grains, legumes, healthy fats, proteins, antioxidants, and nutrients from spices and herbs that empower the core and prevent unhealthy inflammation, which underlies many serious ailments and hinders wellness and longevity. Nutrigenomics, an exciting new field of study that examines the relationship between nutrition and genetics, may one day soon provide us with our own individually-tailored diet plans based on genetic makeup. Advances in digital tools and artificial intelligence will help individuals track nutrient intakes and identify nutritional gaps based on their genetic profiles. This field has great promise for the prevention and treatment of disease.

A plethora of dietary plans purport to provide optimal nutrition, yet scientists agree the majority of our diets should be based on minimally processed foods close to nature, primarily plants. Considering the future well-being of mankind, the majority of our diet must be plant-based to benefit our bodies and the planet, as human health is intricately and inextricably connected to planetary health. The USDA 2020 Dietary Guidelines concur that foods of plant origin are best for human health and the environment alike, recommending that more than 75 percent of dietary intake be of plant origin. Dietary patterns rich in colorful plant foods and limited in animal products favor human health, support belly microbial diversity, and promote planetary health by lowering greenhouse gas emissions.

Women do better on a higher-fat diet than men, with slightly fewer carbohydrates and protein. They burn more fat, but fewer carbohydrates and less protein than men at the same exercise intensity level. Women normally have a higher body fat percentage than men of the same weight, not only on their bodies but also within their muscles, so they use fat as their primary energy source. This means women don't need as many carbohydrates or as much protein to fuel their cores. Fats, in moderation, have positive effects on the hormonal and cardiovascular health of women. Low-fat diets may even reduce breast size, likely due to the low hormone production. A delicious, holistic diet that ensures adequate fat intake is easier to adhere to, so don't deprive yourself of occasional decadent splurges to nourish your body and spirit!

Water for Wellness

> "Water is the driving force of all nature."
> —Leonardo da Vinci

Water is the life source that makes up 60 percent of your body, which needs water to regulate your core body temperature, rid your body of toxins and wastes, and lubricate and cushion your joints. It is the most essential component of each cell in your body. Adequate hydration levels in each of these cells is inextricably linked to your health. Recent evidence reveals a link between inadequate hydration and obesity, chronic disease, and premature death. Inadequate water intake and excessive water loss adversely affect how you feel, how you function, and even how long you will live.

Assuming you eat a healthy diet, mindful attention to your thirst may be sufficient for regulating hydration levels. Although enough water to satisfy your thirst is sensible for short and light activities where sweat loss is low to moderate, following a planned hydration strategy is recommended for longer exercise periods or work in warm temperatures, where sweat loss can be considerable over many hours.

The National Academies of Sciences, Engineering and Medicine recommend drinking eleven and a half cups of fluids each day for women, fifteen and a half cups a day for men, and even more in hot weather or with high activity levels. These recommendations consider both beverages and foods as sources of water, so fruits and vegetables that are high in water content can also count toward that goal. While you're exercising, drink extra water to recover the fluid lost in sweat. As a general guideline, drink a couple of cups of water before exercising, half a cup every fifteen minutes during your training, and at least a couple of cups afterward. Thirst may often be confused with hunger, so be sure to drink when you're feeling hungry too.

We all have distinct physiologies with unique hydration needs based on our size, sweat rate, environment, and hormonal fluctuations. For women, low levels of female hormones during menstruation contribute to dehydration and sap their energy levels. Estrogen is associated with the body's ability to retain water, and the lower it is, the less the body holds onto. This fluctuation may result in an increased risk of dehydration. Blood volume decreases during times of high hormonal levels; therefore, less fluid is available to sweat, inhibiting body temperature regulation. Female hormones also deplete salt, making women more susceptible than males to hyponatremia. Hyponatremia is a rare, potentially life-threatening condition that can affect both females and males, so be vigilant of your sodium dietary intake during long, intense workouts or endurance events, and consume sports drinks that contain electrolytes.

There's no one-size-fits-all formula for avoiding dehydration or overhydration, so it's important to get in tune with your own body's needs. Like a car, your body must dissipate excess heat generated from the fuel you burn when you move or exercise. Unfortunately, there is no dipstick or gauge to tell you how much fluid you have in your system, or when to "add a quart." By the time you feel thirsty, your body may already have lost enough water to impact the function of every cell, tissue, and organ of your body. Even mild dehydration can negatively affect your energy, mood, attention, memory, heart function, and motor coordination. This is particularly important for older adults over sixty-five years old, as the sensation of thirst gets weaker with age, so they don't always realize when they are dehydrated.

Look for signs of dehydration (dark urine, cracked lips, fatigue, dizziness, or sunken eyes) or overhydration (fatigue, dizziness, headache, confusion, muscle cramps, or nausea). Just 1 percent of body fluid loss may cause some sluggishness, whereas 2 to 4 percent (considered mild dehydration) can be detected by reduced and darkened urine. Moderate dehydration (4 to 8 percent fluid loss) makes your skin, lips, and mouth dry. Body fluid loss exceeding 8 percent, considered severe dehydration, causes fever, irritability, and confusion. If loss exceeds 10 percent, body temperature increases and blood pressure decreases, which can be life-threatening.

It's important to cultivate self-awareness of your hydration, how well you recognize your feelings, and where your feelings come from. Discover the right fluid levels for your body to improve your digestion and circulation, promote weight loss, revitalize your hair and skin, prolong your youthful aura, and replenish your core to improve the quantity and quality of your years.

Unplug and Recover

"Disconnecting from our technology
to reconnect with ourselves is absolutely essential."
—Arianna Huffington

Recovery from exercise is just as important as exercise itself. Whether you're exercising to look or feel better, or training for an Ironman triathlon, more isn't always better. A successful program isn't complete without rest days to replenish your energy. Allowing time for your body to recover actually improves performance and decreases the risk of overtraining, burnout, and injury.

When you are overworked, you are more likely to compromise your body's mechanics, whether you take a wrong step or wipe out on your bike. Overtraining also exposes your muscles and tendons to repetitive stress and strain, increasing your risk of fatigue, pain, and overuse injuries. This happens when you train more than your body can recover from to the point that your performance degrades. The most common causes of overtraining are drastic increases in intensity, frequency, and/or duration of your exercise without sufficient time for recovery. Allow your body to recover and repair so you can build stronger muscles by increasing workout intensity gradually and taking breaks. Do not overexert yourself, and make sure you know your limits.

Learning to listen to your body's needs is more important for your progress and improved performance than pushing yourself as hard as you can every day, regardless of your fitness level or sport. Symptoms of overtraining include extreme fatigue, performance decline, and mood disturbances. Recovery of your mind and spirit are equally important for complete wellness. In today's fast-paced world, in which work-life or school-life balance may be challenging, the virtue of hard work is ingrained in our culture. Americans already work more hours per year than their peers around the world. Over the past fifty years, the percentage of working mothers has increased from 20 to 70 percent, and three out of four of these women work full time. Almost all professionals in the United States report working more than fifty hours per week, and nearly half work more than sixty-five hours per week.

We are not only asked to work more, but more is expected of us, as we have increased productivity by 400 percent per worker since

1950, when the stress from a typical eight-hour shift was left at the workplace. Technological advances have heightened expectations of 24/7 accessibility, keeping us plugged in around the clock. Competition at work or school further incentivizes long work hours. The stress from this never-ending workday has a negative impact on our relationships, health, and overall happiness.

Prevent your work from infecting your life by setting boundaries and taking time to unplug. Learn to shut off your phone or computer and enjoy the moment, especially in the evening. Kick the habit of scrolling social media or newsfeeds on your phone, as this increases anxiety and depression, and negatively affects your sleep. Don't allow texts and emails to interrupt your recovery time and cause stress. Creating healthy habits around how you use your phone, computer, TV, and other devices will help you gain a greater sense of control over your life, stay more relaxed, and achieve more of your life.

Spend quality time with your loved ones and pursue your own interests and activities to nourish yourself. After all, a life of only work and sleep is akin to slavery and can be destructive to your entire being. Banish burnout by learning to live in the moment, and tune in to mindful breathing while engaging all of your senses to soak in the universe around you. Make a commitment to reconnect with and nurture your core. Treat yourself to a well-deserved nap, sauna session, or a massage to release all the tension and invigorate your body, mind, and spirit.

Recharge Your Battery

"Sleep is the best meditation."
—Dalai Lama

Sleep nourishes your mind-body-spirit and is integrally related to nutrition and wellness, as Shakespeare recognized hundreds of years ago when he wrote that slumber is the "chief nourisher in life's feast." Sufficient quantity and quality of sleep are equally vital for optimal functioning and homeostasis of all your biological processes, including digestion, immunity, hormonal balance, mental health, learning, memory, clearance of toxins, growth, healing, and cell regeneration.

Most children and teens need at least nine to ten hours of sleep to support growth and development, whereas most adults should ideally sleep seven to eight hours. However, the average American sleeps only four to six hours per night. Sleep loss contributes to a cumulative debt, which impairs the ability of your mind and body to function. Sleeping more on days off from work or school is a sign of sleep deprivation. Although "catching up" may help you feel better, this may also disrupt your body's sleep/wake rhythm and could lead to further sleep problems.

Insufficient sleep increases your levels of stress hormones and may have serious health consequences, such as neurological deficits (in memory, concentration, or neuromuscular control) and cardio-metabolic risks (of heart disease, obesity, diabetes, and infections). When you are sleep deprived, naps improve your attentiveness, coordination, reflexes, and spirit. A twenty-minute snooze enhances motor skills and mental clarity, while fifty to ninety minutes of napping regulates your nervous system and brings deeper REM (Rapid Eye Movement) sleep, which helps you to generate new connections in the brain and core. Sleep is the natural way to recover energy, so you should use naps instead of energy drinks or caffeine when you need a boost.

Dedicating time for adequate restorative sleep protects your health and well-being now and in the future. While your conscious self is off duty, several other systems are hard at work during the night shift. Your night crew is busy repairing your muscles, building your bones, replenishing your energy reserves, and refreshing your nervous system's software. New data is updated from the neuromuscular learning that occurred during the day, and your neural trash is emptied by clearing toxins from your brain.

The nervous system actually reactivates and reorganizes recently learned information, improving muscle memory and boosting performance. Have you ever seen a sleeping puppy mimic running while sound asleep? I remember swooshing and carving down the slope in my own dreams after the first time I learned to snowboard. These are examples of your night crew hard at work to improve your body's functioning. If you want to get better at a skill, you need plenty of sleep for your brain to actually learn to improve. If your unconscious self's night shift is cut short, your body and mind don't have time to adequately recharge and reap all the benefits of everything you learned during the day.

Night after night of insufficient sleep increasingly wears you down mentally and physically, making you more prone to injury. So, make sure you take the time for full recovery to ensure all systems are ready to go. Avoid factors that can disrupt your sleep, such as drinking caffeinated or alcoholic beverages in the evening, or using electronics before bedtime.

There is new research linking the blue light that's emitted from screens to serious health problems such as cancer, diabetes, obesity, heart disease, and vision loss. Blue light also tricks your body into thinking it's daytime, inhibiting the release of melatonin, the hormone that helps you sleep. Instead of looking at a screen before bed, try to establish a relaxing pre-sleep routine, such as a soothing bath, mindful breathing, or meditation. Healthy sleep habits will help you learn faster, get stronger and more fit, and protect yourself from many kinds of diseases.

Nourish Your Soul

"A happy soul has the power to build a healthy body and an intelligent mind."
—Sharath

In traditional Western medicine, focus is placed on the health of the body and the mind, but the "spirit" part, the whole person, is often overlooked. The spiritual dimension is an elusive component of holistic health that is necessary for empowering individuals and populations for wellness and disease prevention. Spirituality, a wide-ranging concept with many perspectives, is a domain of awareness where we experience universality, or a sense of connection to something greater than ourselves. It is a universal human experience, yet it touches all of us in distinctive ways.

For some, a spiritual experience is transcendent, and for others it is a deep sense of vitality and interconnectedness. For many people, spiritual life is intricately linked to their association with a place of worship, whereas others find comfort in a personal relationship with God or a higher power. Still others fill their spirit through their connections with nature, art, or music. Taking time to ponder spiritual questions about your identity and life purpose, exploring connections to the world around you, or seeking a meaningful connection with the universe can create positive emotions such as peace, awe, contentment, gratitude, and acceptance.

A new consciousness of the ageless wisdom of our ancestors is re-emerging in health and wellness. The scientific community is recognizing the bigger picture of health as alchemy between body and soul. True holistic wellness is integrally linked to the inherent power of the human spirit. The World Health Organization acknowledges that the "existing definition of healthcare should include the spiritual" and that "human spirituality is a tightly woven integration of an insightful relationship with yourself and others, a strong personal value system, and the fulfillment of a meaningful purpose to your life."

Abundant research supports spirituality's tangible influence on our bodies and our lives. The benefits of spirituality on mental and physical health include a greater psychological well-being, relief from stress, and decreased immune system proteins associated with age-related diseases. New research also shows that people who attend religious services, or who identify as spiritual, experience lower levels of depression, display signs of better health (such as lower blood pressure and fewer strokes), and claim to feel generally healthier.

Spirituality is a very personal experience, and everyone's spiritual path is unique. Squeezing some relaxation, reflection, contemplation, and meditation into your daily life, even just a few minutes, will foster spiritual wellness and allow you to explore your spiritual core to identify your purpose, your values, and your relationship to the universe around you. Explore your own spiritual stress relief strategies and see what works to nurture, restore, and renew your soul, whether it's getting out in the woods, attending a religious retreat, or climbing Machu Picchu.

Spiritual awakening is important for the state of consciousness with which you meet the world. Recognize the value of spirituality in your life to improve how you cope with the stresses of everyday events and increase your chances of living longer. You should nurture your spirit, no matter what your source of inspiration. Rediscover a forgotten spiritual path or reinforce your commitment to an already well-established one. Be good to your mind-body-spirit and it will be good to you!

Seeds for Thought

- What effects—either positive or negative—do you think your current lifestyle choices have on your core and overall health?

- Are there any changes you'd like to make?

- Do you currently get adequate sleep and drink enough water to stay sufficiently hydrated? If not, make a plan to increase both.

- How will you choose to practice self-care and self-love to nourish your mind-body-spirit?

- What are three things you're grateful for this week? How does it feel to express conscious gratitude?

CHAPTER 8

The Floor of the Core

"If the foundation is firm the building can withstand calamities."
—B.K.S. Iyengar

In 2007, I watched my belly transform from a washboard to a beach ball, to finally what looked like an alien trying to break out. In the late months of my pregnancy, I developed a natural separation down the middle of my abdominal muscles, caused by the stretch and strain from my growing baby. The "alien" was actually the connective tissue between my separated abs, and is really called a "diastasis recti." This is common during and after pregnancy for 60 percent of women (especially in athletes with tight abs), or after a sudden weight gain, and can also happen in men.

The separation causes a protruding belly that can hang around even after returning to normal weight, no matter how many sprints or crunches you do to tone your core. I also demonstrated another tell-tale sign of a compromised core: a diminished ability to speak or sing loudly, or to have a deep, hearty laugh, all of which increase abdominal pressure and can wreak havoc on a stressed core floor. An embattled core post-partum may cause problems for years to come if not corrected. These consequences can include pelvic and back pain, digestive problems, prolapse (the slipping down of your organs), and even death.

As a triathlete, I was motivated to continue my training throughout pregnancy (albeit modified in intensity), and set a new goal to retrain my core so I could run the New York City marathon three months after the birth of my son. I had witnessed patients, friends, and family suffer from post-partum depression, and I needed a goal that would motivate me to get my mind and core back on track. Although my Ob-Gyn recommended surgical correction to repair the split in my abdominal muscles, I used the principles of the Core BASE to slowly but surely retrain my core muscles to reunite and reestablish my stable core.

Having a baby may not only compromise the abdominal muscles, but also the pelvic floor musculature (the sling of muscles and ligaments that stretch from the front pubic bone to the back tailbone) by stretching during pregnancy or tearing during childbirth. This is your core floor, which acts like a hammock to support the undercarriage of your internal organs. Pelvic floor dysfunction, which affects millions of people, is finally being recognized and treated as a serious medical condition that impacts emotional, psychological, and sexual wellness.

A woman's anatomy predisposes her to less support of the pelvic and abdominal organs when compared with a man. The male pelvic floor has a better mechanical advantage, as the female pelvic floor has more organs to hold, plus an extra opening to compromise the integrity of the supporting hammock. This is why it's especially important for women to train their pelvic floor muscles. Pregnancy, childbirth, disuse, overuse, aging, trauma, and weight gain may cause problems for your pelvic floor. This is also very common in athletes who experience the same issue when coughing, holding deep breaths, and performing heavy lifting or high impact exercises. Athletes are at greater risk for pelvic floor issues due to frequent increases in abdominal pressure while training and performing, especially when it comes to jumping and landing.

Years ago, women simply accepted years of incontinence or leaking after childbirth as the price to pay for the miracle of their child. However, pelvic floor dysfunction is no longer the "elephant in the room," as new research and awareness have drawn more attention to this common problem in both women and men. We now know that retraining of the pelvic floor musculature, with postural awareness and core strengthening, is the best way to address the many issues caused by pelvic floor dysfunction. Exercising your pelvic floor muscles probably doesn't cross your mind when you think of an ideal workout routine, yet it should, because a strong core floor will not only help you reduce your risk of developing pelvic floor issues and back pain, but also improve your body image and sexual health, maximize your core strength and stability, and boost your overall wellness.

Deep Breathing to Engage Your Floor and Stabilize Your Core

"Conscious breathing is my anchor."
—Thich Nhat Hanh

Deep breathing helps you get in tune with your pelvic region, a vital center of your body's holistic functioning. Faulty breathing during strenuous movements is a common source of injury. Among the muscles involved in breathing and trunk strengthening, the pelvic floor muscles have long been ignored. Optimal performance is only achieved by connecting your breath and pelvic floor muscle function to all of your movements.

To understand this connection, think about how you hold your breath and suck in your belly when you are dying to go to the bathroom. When you do this, your balloon-shaped abdominal cavity is being compressed by all of your core muscles, including your pelvic floor, the hammock on the bottom of the balloon. The web of pelvic floor muscles works in cooperation with your other core muscles as pressure is generated in this balloon whenever you breathe, talk, or cough.

Contraction of the pelvic floor activates the inner core muscles and is important for protecting internal organs and control of your trunk stability for all activities. When you do something that requires breathing out forcefully, like singing or shouting, your core muscles contract more strongly, increasing the pressure in your abdomen and the pelvic floor muscles, which need to contract to support your organs for postural control, core stability, and continence. This concept underlies the importance of breath training coordinated with the pelvic floor and core activation.

Deep breathing exercises are key for developing pelvic floor activation. Shallow breathing doesn't provide enough oxygen for your muscles and organs, and it doesn't establish the important coordination needed between the pelvic floor and core muscles. If you do not practice deep breathing, then your pelvic floor will stay tense and rigid. When practicing your daily mindful breathing, try to develop an awareness of the lengthening of your core floor (dropping) during the breath in, and the natural elevation of the pelvic floor during the breath out to better understand your own pelvic floor rhythm. You can tune in to this rhythm to relieve anxiety and rid your body of tension and fatigue.

Ocean Breathing

"It's always ourselves we find in the sea."
—E.E. Cummings

Take a deep breath in through your nose, expanding your belly all the way down to your core floor. Then, breathe out through your mouth, making a sound like a giant seashell as you exhale. Imagine fogging a mirror with your breath. With your mouth closed, recreate the same action at the back of your throat by mimicking the sound of the ocean, or the natural sigh you make when you are stressed or worried, to regulate your physical and emotional state. This is one of the best ways to increase awareness and activation of your diaphragm and pelvic floor.

Retrain and tone your diaphragm and core floor in harmony using a slow exhalation pattern. Breathing through pursed lips helps reduce rapid breathing and higher carbon dioxide levels during and after exercise, or during stressful situations that illicit quick, inefficient breathing. You can also imagine blowing through a straw, or blowing slowly and steadily on a candle flame so as to make it flicker but not extinguish.

Try to sigh as loudly and as long as you can, like a balloon expelling air. Imagine your breath coming from deep within your pelvic floor, and carry it through your core to your mouth. Stay connected to the rise and fall of the pelvic floor, staying focused on your breath, which will decrease your fight or flight overactivity and encourage a relaxation response.

Lion's Breath

"It's better to live one day as a lion than a thousand days as a lamb."
—Roman proverb

Lion's breath is a breathing strategy that involves rapid cyclical activation and the release of your core floor to expand lung capacity and promote awareness, mobility, and balance of your core. Your breath is the foundation for helping bring true strength and stability to the pelvic floor. Lion's breath engages and helps to balance the core floor using quick, rhythmic, continuous breaths through the nose, with the mouth closed. Be sure to release all tension from your face, limbs, and trunk. The fast breaths are equal in length on the inhalation and exhalation, with no pause between them.

Seasoned practitioners of Lion's Breath can work up to a rate of approximately two to three cycles per second for one full minute. However, you should listen to your own body and progress your rate slowly, and discontinue the practice if you start to feel lightheaded. With the wave of each breath, your core floor moves like an ocean buoy, rising with the breath out, and falling with the breath in. Focus your attention on this activation and release, or lengthening of the core floor, and prepare your core to engage upon demand.

Healthy pelvic floor function is not just about strength; it is also about the pelvic floor's movement and balance in relation to the core. The goal is to connect your mind to your pelvic floor rhythm through deep breathing. Once you develop the neuromuscular mind-body connection with the fluidity of your pelvic floor movement, you can progress to a more rapid voluntary pelvic floor exercise to enhance your core awareness and learn to control how your body functions and deals with physical and emotional stress.

Try these with your partner to turn up the bedroom heat. It's not only fun, but it's great for connecting in body, mind, and spirit. Practicing the balance of engaging and releasing is essential for finding your center and learning to live from your core. True enlightenment is finding your on/off switch for your core floor and learning to control the dimmer to achieve a flat tummy, great sex, and a healthy, powerful body.

In Eastern health and medicine, the core floor is called the root chakra, or "muladhara" in Sanskrit, with "mula" meaning "root" and "adhara" meaning "support" or "base." Your core floor is the root of what grounds you to true stability. A solid physical and metaphysical foundation of your core base will embed your core in firm soil to provide the stability you need to truly flourish. The Core BASE Guide will teach you how to establish this foundation through mindful meditation, dynamic stretching for alignment and balance, and core activation, strengthening, and stabilization.

"Laughing So Hard That You Pee" Isn't So Funny

"You can only solve a problem which you recognize to be a problem."
—R.G. Collingwood

A weak pelvic floor can cause you to leak while laughing, exercising, sneezing, coughing, bending, lifting, or jumping. These activities create pressure in your abdomen, which can result in a failure to hold your pee (or worse!). This is an indication that the coordinated movement of the pelvic floor is disrupted. Muscles may be too tight (not relaxed enough) or too weak (not contracted enough). Urinary incontinence is a health problem that affects the quality of millions of lives at all stages.

According to recent data, the incidence of urinary incontinence ranges from 30 to 70 percent in women and up to 15 percent in men. This is a distressful issue that affects both sexes and can not only damage your self-esteem, but lead to depression, anxiety, and yield negative repercussions for your sex life and overall quality of life. Many factors can weaken your core floor, including pregnancy, childbirth, surgery, aging, straining, and weight gain. Some may think this is a normal part of aging, and many are too embarrassed to seek help.

Because the core floor works in coordination with all of your core musculature, recent studies show that incorporating pelvic floor muscle training with synergistic core activation is more effective at improving bladder control than pelvic floor exercises alone. Activating your core floor elevates the pressure in your belly and elicits coactivation of all your core muscles that act together as a team. The Core BASE Guide will show you how to incorporate these simple exercises into your daily routine so you can gain control and prevent embarrassing accidents.

Most people have heard of "Kegel" exercises, yet many do not know how to perform them correctly. These simple exercises involve squeezing and relaxing your pelvic floor to enhance your core floor tone. Toning of your undercarriage improves bladder control, sexual function, and control of your core, and is important for both women and men! One of the keys to keeping your floor strong is learning how to find and engage it.

Core Floor Toning

"Tell me and I'll forget. Show me and I'll remember. Involve me and
I'll learn."
—Benjamin Franklin

Learning to engage your core floor requires daily, diligent practice.
Imagine your pelvic floor as a diamond-shaped sling of muscles that
supports your core and stops urination mid-stream; that's the area you
want to target during core floor toning. Breathe in and relax your core
floor, then breathe out as you activate your core floor. When you breathe
out or speak, your core floor automatically contracts, making the muscle
activation stronger. Breathe out as you contract your pelvic floor muscles,
then relax your core floor muscles again on your inhalation.

A contraction of the core floor results in a constriction and inward
movement of the pelvic openings. Squeeze and lift your core floor
by imagining you are trying to stop your pee mid-flow. A visual of
squeezing and lifting a marble into the vagina helps most women
learn to activate these muscles. For men, imagine walking into a cold
ocean, drawing your "boys to your belly" as the freezing water hits your
thighs. For both men and women, constricting the anus, as if to prevent
passing gas, is also a helpful cue for activating the core floor. Try this in
front of a hand mirror. If performed properly, women should see the
area between the vagina and anus contract and lift, and men should
see the base of the penis draw in and scrotum lift up. Focus on toning
only your pelvic floor muscles with your glutes relaxed to improve your
focused awareness and connection with your core floor. Breathe freely
during the exercises, and avoid holding your breath. Holding your
breath pushes down on the core floor, which is trying to lift up. That
means your body is fighting itself.

There are two important variations of the core floor toners:
quickies and endurance exercises. Make sure to practice quickie core
floor toners by contracting and lifting your core floor for one to two
seconds, but be sure to also mix in some endurance exercises by holding
for as long as you can, maintaining your core floor tone as you breathe.

Make both types of contractions part of your daily routine, as
both are beneficial, since the pelvic floor is comprised of two types of
muscle fibers: fast and slow.

Fast muscle fibers provide quick activation, efficiency, and power to the core floor. When focusing on the fast fibers, make sure to activate your core floor quickly, and then fully release in between contractions. Use deep, mindful breathing to ensure all the other muscles of your body remain relaxed.

Endurance core floor toning targets your slow muscle fibers to build muscle stamina in these important core-stabilizing muscles. Contract the pelvic floor muscles and hold this contraction for as long as you can, working towards at least ten seconds. Again, make sure to relax completely in between each repetition, as the relaxation of your floor is just as important as the tightening. This is an important principle to understand for the pelvic floor, but also with any other type of exercise. Be patient with your floor, as it may take weeks or months for full benefits to be realized.

Just like all of your core muscles, stability is achieved through muscle strength, endurance, and timing. In a healthy core floor, turning the muscles on is a reflexive action that kicks in when you need it, such as when you cough, sneeze, jump, or lift something heavy. Once you get the knack of these exercises, you can work on the rhythm and timing of your core floor contraction. However, if you've lost your connection with your core floor, this reflexive contraction may be lost too. With diligent practice, this connection can be re-established with a strong and well-timed contraction to regain your confidence in potentially embarrassing moments.

Tone your pelvic floor for better strength, endurance, and timing by lying on your back, before progressing to sitting, and then standing. Eventually, you should incorporate these practices into any movements of your daily life, such as while you are watering your garden, washing your car, riding your bike, or having fun with your partner for some sexercise!

Don't Just Tighten, Enlighten

"Knowing others is wisdom, knowing yourself is enlightenment."
—Lao Tzu

The release phase of your core floor toning exercises is just as critical as the tightening phase. A full squeeze and full relax constitutes one repetition. Over-clenching can shorten the muscles of your pelvic floor. A tight, unrelaxed pelvic floor occurs when the muscles in the pelvic floor become too tense. This may cause constipation, urgency to pee, or pelvic pain. Too much core floor tone can also increase your risk of leaking, make it more difficult to achieve orgasm, or even cause painful sex.

If you work out often with heavy weights, or keep your core muscles engaged all the time, you may also develop too much tension in your core floor by keeping these muscles switched on without some time to relax. Many people try to keep their tummies flat by sucking in the abdomen to give the illusion of a trim figure, but this habit pulls down the abdominal contents, compresses the organs, and applies downward pressure, creating more tension on the core floor and forcing it to work overtime.

If you have the habit of holding it in when you feel the need to go to the bathroom, you may also develop tension in your pelvic floor muscles. Many people feel uncomfortable using an unfamiliar bathroom and will wait hours (or even days) until they are back home. This means the pelvic floor muscles are tightening to prevent loss of control. Birth trauma scarring may also contribute to core floor tightness, which, combined with "sucking it in" to trim your figure after childbirth, puts the core floor under tremendous pressure. Tight pelvic muscle tone and reduced capacity to stretch reduces the flow of blood and oxygen to your muscles and organs. This creates an unhealthy, acidic environment, which may cause pain and inflammation.

Jaw-Dropping Link

"We cannot direct the wind, but we can adjust the sails."
—Dolly Parton

The connection between your core floor and your jaw begins in the third week of embryonic development, when they are joined by your spine. From this time on, the jaw and pelvis are strongly linked in mind-body-spirit, as tensions in the two areas very often mirror each other. The pelvic floor is integrally linked with your entire being, which includes your emotions and nervous system.

Emotions such as fear, anger, and stress can cause you to reflexively clench and develop tension and tightness in both the jaw and pelvic floor, as well as all other parts of your body. Just as a frightened puppy runs away with its tail between its legs, humans have a primitive response during fight or flight where the tailbone tucks under, causing the core floor muscles to shorten. The core floor is a major stress bucket for your body!

Women in particular tend to internalize emotions more often, which manifests as muscle tension in an unrelaxed core floor. When muscles tense, they constrict the nerves that send electrical signals between your muscles and your brain, causing spasms, weakness, and/or pain. Muscle tension also compromises blood flow, which deprives your muscles of the vital oxygen and nutrients they need to function optimally.

Most people do not even realize that they cruise through much of their day "riding their clutch," with the core floor engaged all the time. When new drivers learn how to shift gears, it takes practice to get the hang of fully disengaging and re-engaging the clutch. This causes mechanical problems in a car, just as having a constantly engaged core floor does in your body. If you never fully disengage your core floor, you may experience tightness, decreased range of motion, and even pain. Awareness and mindful relaxation of tense muscles is the key to good nerve transmission and blood circulation, which is necessary for a healthy core floor. Again, this takes practice!

To practice relaxation of your core floor, scan your body for areas of tension and gently release, as you practice your mindful deep breathing. Gently place your tongue behind your front teeth to relax your jaw and think of something that makes you happy and grateful. Fully relax your pelvic floor with each inhalation. If you tense up your pelvic floor muscles, you'll notice that your jaw will also tighten up. Relax one, and the other will follow.

Visualization helps relax the floor, so think of a peaceful place such as a mountain, forest, or beach. Imagine what you would see, hear, feel, smell, and taste, and let your floor go. Reconnect with your pelvic floor to stop driving through life riding your clutch, and cruise your way to a relaxed and balanced core, mind, and life.

Connecting the Pieces

"Dem Bones"

"Your toe bone's connected to your foot bone.
Your foot bone's connected to your heel bone.
Your heel bone's connected to your ankle bone.
Your ankle bone's connected to your leg bone.
Your leg bone's connected to your knee bone.
Your knee bone's connected to your thigh bone.
Your thigh bone's connected to your hip bone
Your hip bone's connected to your back bone
Your back bone's connected to your shoulder bone.
Your shoulder bone's connected to your neck bone.
Your neck bone's connected to your head bone
Now, hear the word of the Lord.
Dem bones, dem bones gonna walk around!"
—James Weldon Johnson

We used to sing this spirited chorus during Anatomy lab as we dissected cadavers. Back then, I had no idea just how resonant this song would turn out to be in my future quest for injury prevention throughout my career. I remember singing this song with such enthusiasm after I aced my final exam and was invited to be the assistant professor for the next year's class.

In retrospect, it's funny to think how confident I was in my knowledge of the human body as a young student, not recognizing how much there still was (and is) to learn. As the great thinkers realized thousands of years ago, "true wisdom comes to each of us when we realize how little we understand about life, ourselves, and the world around us" (Socrates) and, "the more you know, the more you realize you don't know" (Aristotle).

When I graduated three decades ago, the injury rate disparity between the sexes, particularly in knee injuries, was just beginning to be investigated, with a convergence of studies recognizing a significantly higher rate of injury in females than in males, which spurred international collaboration and significant government funding to help solve this tremendous problem.

My quest for answers to this dilemma began with a focused lens on the knee. I started researching the muscle and ligament imbalances of the knock-kneed collapse seen in female sports injuries. Since the knee bone is connected to the hip bone, my graduate research moved on up the chain to the hip, where we recognized altered gluteal posterior chain activation in female athletes, associated with the knee-collapsing injury mechanism. The hip bone is connected to the trunk, where we next turned, and found our groundbreaking correlation between impaired core awareness and impaired core control, which is now an important part of injury prevention programs for athletes worldwide.

It's fitting that this song has spiritual connotations, as we are now recognizing that our chain does not end in our bodies, but continues with our minds and spirits. This exciting paradigm is widening our lens of true holistic wellness and injury prevention by acknowledging the alchemy between all aspects of humanity and spirituality, including the inherent power of the body, mind, and soul and our inextricable link with the universe. After all, isn't everything connected to the "universe bone"? Now that you understand the fundamental concepts of core holistic wellness, it's time to master your own core perception for true empowerment with the Core BASE Guide!

Seeds for Thought

- Do you currently suffer from any issues related to a dysfunctional core floor, such as incontinence, lower back pain, prolapse (bladder, uterine, or bowel), or compromised sexual health?

- Do you often catch yourself feeling tense, or "riding your clutch" throughout your day? In what kinds of situations do you notice it most often?

- During which daily routines do you think you can integrate working on your core floor?

- How did the mindful body scan feel? Did it help to release tension?

- Did you notice the connection between a tense jaw and tense pelvic floor muscles?

PART 2. THE CORE BASE GUIDE

"What you need to do is build the house you will live in. You build that house by laying a solid foundation: by building physical, emotional, mental, and spiritual health."
—James Altucher

The Core BASE Guide outlines the steps you need to develop and improve the perception, activation, and strength of your core while dramatically improving the way you feel, move, and look. You'll learn how to establish your mind-core connection with your breath, restore your body's optimal alignment, decrease tension in your muscles and your nervous system, and maximize your flexibility, strength, and power. Deep breathing, dynamic stretching, and evidence-based core awareness and empowering exercises will be described and illustrated in detail, including modifications and progressions for all ability levels.

You'll also find scientific guidelines to establish your "base" for a leaner, stronger, more powerful body and a healthier, happier mind. Using the power of your breath and 50 core-empowering exercises, you'll be on your way to transforming your body so it can move more effectively with a stable and centered feeling. Activities like bending, turning, reaching, lifting, gardening, or work-related tasks such as prolonged sitting, standing, or walking will all be easier and safer with a stable core. The BASE will also teach you to augment core power and control for the more challenging athletics that you currently enjoy or would love to try (such as marathons, racket sports, golfing, kayaking, paddle-boarding, skiing/snowboarding, or your favorite exercise class) with less fear of injury.

You're about to learn how to improve your health, reduce your risk of injuries, and become functionally fit by using science-based movements that will challenge you with balance exercises, medicine balls, instability devices, plyometrics and suspension training, teaching your body to be ready for anything life throws at you with a heightened level of awareness, stability and confidence. You'll also learn about some of the alternative philosophies and activities that are scientifically proven to harness your energy for core empowerment through Pilates, yoga, martial arts, dance, music, laughter, and nature to build your core foundation and achieve optimal physical, emotional, mental, and spiritual health.

4 Phases of the Core BASE Guide

The Core BASE Guide is broken down into four key phases to help you develop proper core awareness, stability, and control from a solid foundation. Although you may be tempted to skip ahead, I highly recommend you go through all of the exercises of each phase and notice the significant improvement from them before advancing to the next phase. This will help ensure that you develop the proprioception and awareness necessary to perform the more advanced exercises safely and effectively. Jumping past the breathing exercises and heading straight to plyometrics might seem like an exciting idea for an athlete or fitness enthusiast, but you might actually slow your progress by trying to rush the process. So, to get the very best results for your body, I recommend you follow the guide in order.

I also want to reiterate that these exercises are guidelines and not gospel. Some exercises may be too difficult or exhausting for you at first. You should listen to your body and immediately stop any movement that is causing you pain or excessive fatigue, and consult with your healthcare professional. No scientist, physical therapist, or author knows your body better than you do, so you must learn to be your own ultimate guide on this journey to better health and fitness, and that starts with listening to your own body, noticing what you feel, and making adjustments when something isn't working for you.

Breathing:

You'll learn to breathe deeply with dynamic stretches
to align, awaken, and balance your inner core.

Awareness:

You'll develop a heightened awareness of your mind-core connection
through meditation and core exercises for activation, strength, and
coordination.

Stability:

You'll improve the stability of your core with functional exercises that
will challenge your core control and dynamic alignment.

Empowerment:

You'll learn to empower your core using principles of ancient wisdom
and modern science to unleash your full potential from within to feel
more centered, positive, and powerful.

CHAPTER 9

Breathing

"The mind is the king of the senses, but the breath is the king
of the mind."
—Svatmarama

Let's start your path to core empowerment by learning to breathe
deeply and connect your mind with your core. As James Joyce wrote,
"There is no past, no future; everything flows in an eternal present." If
you don't make self-care a priority in your life, you will pay a very high
price as your health declines. Take time every day to fully experience
the present moment, awaken your senses, and establish effective and
efficient mindful breathing strategies for optimal core activation.

Deep breathing, in combination with the targeted trunk-
stretching exercises you'll learn in this chapter, will help you deepen
your mind-core connection. This is the critical first step to improving
your core health. As you do these exercises, pay special attention to
your breathing and the sensations in your body as you move. Putting
your focus and awareness on your muscles and body is a key step in
improving proprioception and core awareness. Do not rush through
these exercises just to "check them off your list." You will get the
best results by taking your time and focusing on every step of the
process. Experience what it feels like as your muscles engage and move
throughout every part of these exercises. Breath training will increase
the recruitment of core musculature, improve functional biomechanics,
and create new neural connections throughout your brain and body, all
of which will protect and empower you.

Breathing Mechanics

"For breath is life, so if you breathe well you will live long on earth."
—Sanskrit Proverb

Scientific evidence shows us that developing breathing mechanics in coordination with the core musculature (including abdominal and back musculature, as well as the inner core muscles) is important for postural control, core stability, and optimal wellness. Muscles that play important roles in core stability include the diaphragm (the dome-shaped muscles at the base of the lungs) as the superior boundary of the core, the pelvic floor (the muscular sling at the base of your abdomen) as the inferior boundary, the multifidus (which stabilizes the spinal column), and the transverse abdominis (the circumferential boundary) (Figure 7). These muscular boundaries of your trunk work together in unison to produce a corset-like stabilization effect for your core. It is the goal of core stability exercises to activate these respiratory and postural muscles in a coordinated manner, and to maximize 360 degrees of control for complex daily maneuvers and athletic activities.

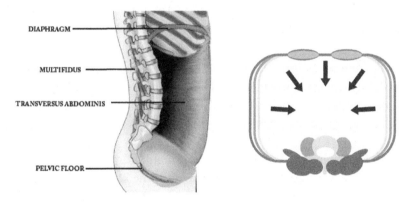

DIAPHRAGM

MULTIFIDUS

TRANSVERSUS ABDOMINIS

PELVIC FLOOR

Figure 7. Inner core muscular boundaries, which contract to produce "corset-like" stabilization, like when you tighten a belt. Diaphragm, Transverse Abdominis, Multifidus and Pelvic Floor. Reprinted with permission from Zazulak BT, Medvecky MJ. Trunk stability for Injury Prevention: The Core of Evidence. CT Medicine. Oct 2019;83(9):443-450.

Diaphragmatic breathing (deep breathing that fully contracts the diaphragm muscle) must be established prior to progressing to more advanced core-empowering exercises. As the superior boundary of the abdomen, the diaphragm increases abdominal pressure by moving downward when it contracts, and facilitates co-contraction of the pelvic floor muscles. Deep breathing patterns provide a stable core with abdominal support around the entire spine, which is critical for injury prevention and your capacity for daily activities and exercise. Breathing is like any movement pattern that can be trained with activation-based strategies to become habitual.

Although ancient cultures have advocated the physiological and psychological benefits of slow, deep breathing on the respiratory, cardiovascular, musculoskeletal, and nervous systems for thousands of years, scientists have only recently jumped on board. The normal respiratory rate is within the range of ten to twenty breaths per minute. Practicing deep diaphragmatic breathing regularly at a rate of four to ten breaths per minute will help improve your health and longevity. Initially, a conscious focus on breathing must be emphasized when any form of stress is placed on the body to get the feeling of how your core engine runs. This conscious preparation will become subconscious over time.

Your Core Engine

"The human body is the magazine of inventions, the patent office, where are the models from which every hint is taken. All the tools and engines on earth are only extensions of its limbs and senses."
—Ralph Waldo Emerson

The diaphragm, the intersection of multiple systems of your body (nervous, musculoskeletal and respiratory), is the key player of your core engine and an easily accessible gateway to controlling your mind-body-spirit. This primary muscle of inspiration forms the floor of the chest under your lungs, and has attachments to the ribs, breastbone, and spine, with neural connections to your mouth, pelvic floor, and heart. When you breathe in, the dome of the diaphragm leads the charge and engages your inner core by contracting downwards into the abdomen, allowing the lungs to expand while increasing abdominal pressure.

When you exhale, your diaphragm relaxes and ascends back to its resting state. A relaxed exhale requires very little effort, as it is the result of the passive recoil of the diaphragm. However, the abdominal muscles can help facilitate a deeper exhalation by narrowing and depressing your rib cage.

In addition to the diaphragm, the rib muscles assist lung expansion by creating space in the rib cage; but, the vast majority of lung expansion that occurs while you breathe happens in the space created by the diaphragm. The efficiency of the diaphragm is deeply connected to the alignment of the rib cage. When the ribs are stacked above the hips, the diaphragm rests in its natural state and has room to move. When the ribs are in a flared or displaced position, the diaphragm is not in its optimal position to facilitate deep inhalation.

As a result, the neck muscles attempt to assist with inhalation by elevating the upper ribs. This leads to neck and shoulder tension, and can limit shoulder mobility by changing the way your shoulder blades are positioned relative to your rib cage. This also inhibits the automatic engagement of the core, leading to postural instability. Similar to the game of Jenga, when all of the blocks are aligned, the tower is stable; however, if the blocks are pulled out of alignment with the tower, stability is lost. The same is true for the body. When the trunk is out of alignment with the pelvis, the posture is not stable, the diaphragm is struggling to assist with postural stability, and breathing becomes shallow and strained.

Apical breathers, or chest breathers, demonstrate exaggerated chest rise and upper rib expansion, rather than diaphragmatic expansion, to increase space for the lungs. This dysfunctional breathing pattern creates reliance on the rib muscles to make room in the chest, and limits the total breath capacity and core stability. To check if you are a chest breather, place one hand on your chest and the other hand on your belly. Take some normal breaths and pay attention to which hand moves more during your inhalation. If you notice that your upper hand moves more, you are a chest breather. Next, wrap your hands around your last few ribs, with thumbs in back and fingers wrapped around the front. This time, take full, deep breaths and pay close attention to your ribs as you breathe in. You should feel your ribs expand into your hands laterally and into your back as well. The diaphragm descends during an inhale, which fills the lungs, expands the ribs, and activates your core muscles.

Stretch Out the Turtle and Catch a Deep Breath!

"In, out.
Deep, slow.
Calm, ease.
Smile, release.
Present moment,
wonderful moment."
—Thich Nhat Hanh

One great way to facilitate diaphragmatic breathing mechanics while checking for excessive chest expansion is to practice deep breathing from your belly. All that time spent on computers and phones leads to a flexed "turtle" posture, which can cause your breath to get stuck high up in your chest, or even your throat. Encourage deeper diaphragmatic breathing mechanics by hopping on your belly for a few minutes a day, morning and night, to improve your postural alignment and reinforce efficient breathing mechanics and core activation. Place your hands on top of each other, resting your forehead on the back of your hands to lift and open your chest.

Breathe deeply into your lower abdomen. Imagine the air filling deep into your belly, and focus on the rise of your lower back before your upper back rises. Picture the air filling you deep down into your core floor and lifting your turtle shell off your back. As this occurs, your lower abdomen will expand into the ground, providing feedback to activate your inner core. You should feel minimal expansion of your chest into the ground. Slow your breath and lengthen your exhalations. With each exhalation, you should feel a gentle squeeze from the sides, front, and base of your abdomen as it expands in 360 degrees. This is a great warm-up exercise to encourage proper breathing mechanics prior to your workouts.

Long-term shallow breathing may actually keep your body in a cycle of stress, detrimentally affecting your mind and body. The stress response of the body is also known as the "fight or flight" response of the sympathetic nervous system. This response is important when confronting danger, and helpful in situations which require us to rise to challenges. However, this response becomes problematic when it is provoked by less momentous situations, and can contribute to a cascade of events that are detrimental to your mind-body-spirit.

Don't Sweat the Small Stuff!

"Out of the clutter, find simplicity. From discord, find harmony."
—Albert Einstein

Excessive activation of the sympathetic nervous system contributes to many health problems, including high blood pressure, immune system suppression, anxiety, depression, digestive disorders, muscle tension, and a shallow breathing pattern, which further compromises posture, body mechanics, and core stability. Inefficient breathing will not only stress the nervous system, but may contribute to headaches, pelvic floor dysfunction, vocal cord pathologies, and other musculoskeletal problems. The consequence of inefficient breathing is a negative feedback cycle in which we begin to over-breathe and rarely make a full exhale.

To counter this in times of stress, breathe through your nose and lengthen your exhalations relative to your inhalations. Work up to a ratio in which you exhale twice as long as you inhale. Lengthening your exhalations will help calm your nervous system (as happens naturally when you sigh) and engage your core muscles to help you feel more centered. Mindful core diaphragmatic breathing calms the sympathetic nervous system and invokes the parasympathetic nervous system (or relaxation response), which reduces stress, anxiety, anger, and inflammation, and is the most important bodily function to supply all cells and organs with oxygen for optimal health.

The autonomic nervous system (which is comprised of the sympathetic and parasympathetic) is also called "involuntary," as it works in a mostly unconscious way to control the vital body function of your breathing, as well as your heart rate, swallowing, digestion, and arousal. But while it mostly functions unconsciously, you do have the power to reset and regulate your autonomic nervous system by extending your exhalations while breathing. So, take an extra second or two to fully expel all of your breath when seeking calm throughout your day, or before sleeping to trigger the relaxation response and to fully engage and balance your inner core muscles, including the diaphragm, multifidus, transverse abdominis, and pelvic floor.

Deep, active, and engaged breathing into the belly activates the core floor musculature. This pelvic floor musculature creates a diamond-shaped frame for the core floor. Proper breathing, which is imperative for healthy pelvic floor function, is analogous to an engine cylinder. On inhalation, the diaphragm (like an engine piston) pushes the abdominal contents down to the pelvic floor. A strong pelvic floor stretches as you breathe in, elastically loads, and contracts as the breath goes up and out. Diaphragmatic motion, combined with recoil and contraction of the pelvic floor musculature, correlate with more effective breathing and are critical for core stabilization.

Until recently, the significance of pelvic floor dysfunction has been underappreciated, with a high incidence of urinary incontinence being underreported. The pelvic floor has long been targeted in the battle against incontinence, and yet it is largely ignored as a critical component of a healthy core. Urinary incontinence indicates decreased inner core control and compromised stability during functional movement. The pelvic floor is a critical part of the inner core squad, and collectively this squad of MVPs works together with all of your core team muscles to keep your center anchored.

High-impact activities increase your risk of pelvic floor dysfunction, but you can counteract the risk with proper core training. Activities such as jumping and running place increased stress on the pelvic floor. Inner core training is effective at improving pelvic floor function and decreasing risk of injury. Integrated teamwork of the core muscles, linked to the up and down piston action of your breath, provides a stable foundation that supports all functional movement.

Blow as You Go!

"As the breath moves, so does the mind, and the mind ceases to move
as the breath is stopped."
—Ancient Indian Parable

Many people tend to facilitate core stability by holding their breath, especially when they exercise, using a technique called the Valsalva Maneuver. This involves exhaling while keeping the glottis (your airway between the vocal folds, which remains open during healthy breathing) closed. A simple comparison for understanding this concept is a tube of toothpaste analogy: when the top is closed, the pressure inside maintains the integrity of the tube, and allows it to withstand outside pressure when you squeeze it. However, when you pop the top open, the pressure inside is diminished, allowing you to easily crush it.

Similarly, holding your breath is a common way to compensate for insufficient core activation during strenuous activities. When you hold your breath, you are closing your airway to increase intra-abdominal pressure in an attempt to compensate for a lack of core stability. This faulty, dangerous breathing strategy becomes especially problematic when the body begins to rely on this method to overcome any stress that is placed on it to make up for inadequate trunk control during simple movements. The glottal hold maneuver imposes negative effects on your cardiovascular system, including increased blood pressure, heart rate, and risk of stroke. Inefficient breathing also deprives your core of fuel, and creates muscular imbalances and adaptations that predispose you to injury.

Linking your breath to your core activation begins with consciously blowing, or exhaling, as you go. This means initiating exhalation prior to movement to trigger a reflexive inner core muscle activation response. Tapping into your inner core reflexive neural response will center you in preparation for all movements or challenges that come your way. With practice, this conscious activation strategy will become natural over time, and you won't have to actually stop and think about it. Functional, coordinated breathing patterns dissociate the breathing cycle from your ability to maintain core stability.

In addition, using mental imagery of breathing mechanics trains the neural circuitry of your core software, but also your core hardware. For instance, an injured javelin athlete can actually minimize muscle loss during recovery by visualizing themselves throwing. Even elderly, wheelchair-bound people can improve their strength by watching yoga videos and imagining themselves doing the exercises. The stronger the image, the more strongly your body will respond. It's amazing that you can actually use your brain to help make you buff with positive visualization! Use your thoughts to redefine the strength and shape of your body.

The Inner Core Toner

"True teaching is not accumulation of knowledge; it is an awakening of consciousness."
—African proverb

Ladies and gentlemen, are you ready to start your core engines? The first and most essential exercise on your path to empowerment is the Inner Core Toner. Think of this more like learning a language rather than exercising. It is impossible to strengthen muscles that your brain cannot activate, so first you must "find" your inner core to activate it properly. Through deep diaphragmatic breathing, you'll activate and strengthen your inner core muscles to create a solid foundation for movement.

The transverse abdominis, one of the key inner core muscles, plays an important role in core stability. The transverse abdominis acts as a deep, muscular corset that wraps all the way around your trunk from your spine to the front of your body, covering your entire torso from breastbone to pubic bone. The fibers of the transverse abdominis are horizontal and decrease the volume of the abdomen in synchrony with your diaphragm, multifidus, and core floor muscles when contracted. This pressurizes your torso, protecting your spine from injurious loads. That's why training your inner core muscles in harmony with your breath is essential.

You can learn to activate your inner core muscles by monitoring the firmness of your transverse abdominis, as this muscle works together with your inner core squad. You can feel this deep muscle contract in the area between your hip bones and just outside of your rectus abdominis, or "six-pack muscle." To check for proper inner core activation, place your hands on your hips and feel the pointy parts of your pelvis under your fingertips. Slide your fingertips slightly inward and downward off the bones. As you tone your belly, you should feel a firmness there. This is an important gauge that can help you check for activation of your inner core squad of muscles.

When first learning to engage your inner core, it is easiest to begin in a hook lying position by lying on your back with your knees comfortably bent and your spine in its neutral, natural alignment (with a gentle curve in your lower back). Take a deep, diaphragmatic inhale through your nose, allowing your abdomen to expand and activate the inner core, completely filling your lungs with air from bottom to top. Imagine breathing into your belly first, then your rib cage, and finally your upper chest as you smile wide with your collar bones.

As you breathe out through your nose, slowly exhale from bottom to top (belly first, then ribcage, then chest). Imagine simultaneously squeezing and lifting up your core floor, slightly drawing circumferentially in your belly button towards your spine, and tightening around the entire trunk circumferentially like a corset (Figure 8). Try to initiate the movement from deep inside the inner core instead of sucking in your stomach, which will actually reduce the stability of your spine. Do not flatten your back, squeeze your glutes, or press the small of your back into the ground; such improper contraction will only activate the superficial muscles, and not the deeper, inner core musculature.

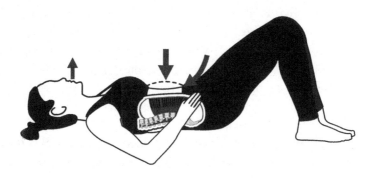

Figure 8. The Inner Core Toner, which involves drawing the inner core muscles up and in while exhaling.

To increase tone, imagine scooping your hip bones together as if they were to kiss one another by contracting your muscles, while simultaneously drawing in your core floor toward your navel. At the end of your exhalations, purse your lips as if breathing through a straw, directing your full effort to your inner core muscles to expel all the air. You should feel your diaphragm, pelvic floor, transversus abdominis, and multifidus activating.

Consciously focus your mind on your inner corset (or abdominal girdle). If you notice your glutes clenching, try to relax them, because tightening them may tilt your lower back out of its natural neutral alignment. To ramp up your core activation, place a strap or band around your lower ribs for resistance and feedback, driving your breath to your belly first, then the strap at your ribs, then your chest.

You must also learn to control your core independently of your breathing; otherwise, your spine may become unstable and more susceptible to injury with every breath. As you get the feel for activating your inner core, you can start working toward maintaining the contraction as you breathe in and out by practicing recruitment in different positions with different activities throughout your day, like waiting at a traffic light or standing in line at a store. This way, you can simultaneously check both your posture and the natural curves of your spine.

Tuning in to the natural engagement of your inner core muscles with your breath will help improve and support your posture throughout all your activities. Although ideally your brain should be telling your core to gently activate during those activities, sometimes your core is tired, weak, or lazy. By consciously activating your core prior to performing those activities, you are retraining your brain and body to protect your spine. Eventually, your brain will take over and activate your core automatically before you begin the activity. Inner core toning will become second nature to you, and the tone of your core should remain steady with each deep breath and prepare you to meet the functional demands of every task.

As the initial exercise and building block of the Core Base Guide, the Inner Core Toner will help you identify and correct abnormal core muscle recruitment. If you struggle with this exercise, that means you really do need further mind-core training until you can achieve solid core muscle tone on command. Just like the core floor toners, you should practice both quickies and endurance variations. Practicing inner core toners of one to two seconds will help you develop the fast pulse of contraction necessary for quick, unexpected perturbations and movements that you'll encounter in everyday life and sports, whereas holding for as long as you can (working up to at least ten seconds) will help train these muscles for sustained activity.

Several weeks of daily training with at least ten repetitions a day may be necessary for this cognitive phase of core stability training, which focuses on improving the sensation and perception of core stability. Most people don't consciously activate their inner core muscles, so it may take some time for you to feel these muscles in action. The ability to perceive activation and relaxation of your inner core musculature improves with repeated practice.

Using this technique to contract your inner core muscles synergistically is essential in order to benefit from core strengthening exercises. This is your first step to establishing your mind-core foundation for core stability and the more advanced exercises of the

Core BASE Guide. This BASE will help you bridge your conscious and unconscious control of your core so you can incorporate automatic and reflexive action into all of your daily activities, whether you're doing household chores or enjoying your favorite dance class.

Motion Is Lotion

"Iron rusts from disuse; stagnant water loses its purity . . . we must stretch ourselves to the very limits of human possibility."
—Leonardo Da Vinci

Stillness is stagnation. Once efficiency of the core engine cylinder is established through mindful diaphragmatic breathing and inner core activation, it's time for a tune-up and oil change. Core-empowering stretches must be incorporated with the power of your breath to lubricate your joints and prepare your core for activity. Stretching is important for health and injury prevention because it increases your joints' range of motion, muscle flexibility, circulation and the elimination of toxins. It also replenishes oxygen and nutrients to fuel your core. Daily stretching of the joints circulates fluid within them, which provides nutrients to cartilage and promotes the release of enkephalins and endorphins, your body's natural pain and stress fighters.

Many researchers have investigated various methods and techniques to determine the most effective ways to stretch. Despite the numerous studies conducted over the past one hundred years, there's still controversy within the scientific community regarding the best methods and techniques for stretching. Clinical research studies support the importance of active (dynamic) stretching with movement to increase muscle flexibility, while others support passive (static) stretching in a fixed position to reduce stiffness and pain. Recent evidence supports a combination of dynamic and static stretches, or massaging with movement, for optimal functioning of your core muscles and nerves to activate and enhance body awareness. Dynamic movements enhance blood flow and stimulate your musculoskeletal and nervous systems, promoting activation and awareness of your core and all its neural connections.

Your nerves are the communication lines between all the muscles of your body, core, and brain. Restricted nerve mobility can lead to pain and potential injury. Poor posture, lack of stretching, and prolonged sitting inhibit the mobility of your peripheral nerves (which run down your arms and legs, and through your muscles on their way from your core to your fingers and toes). When you keep your body in the same posture for prolonged periods, both your nerves and your muscles are shortened.

The nervous system remembers this shortened length and becomes stuck to the tissues of your body. Neural adhesions are common in athletes, especially in sports with repetitive movements, such as baseball, tennis, swimming, and golf. Once a nerve becomes shortened or restricted, it is pulled and irritated over time and may cause numbness, tingling, burning or cold sensations, heaviness, weakness, or altered reflexes. Dynamic stretching will promote gliding and optimal functioning of your nerves, prevent adhesion, encourage optimal information relay to and from your muscles, and keep your nerves healthy as you age.

Deep, active, and engaged breathing, in combination with dynamic and sustained stretches performed at least three times per week, will prepare your core for optimal empowerment. The core dynamic stretches rhythmically shorten and lengthen your muscles, stretching one way and then the other, just as animals innately pandiculate. These dynamic movements stretch the core through cyclic motions (moving further with each repetition toward end range), train your core muscles for optimal activation, and prepare your body for whatever challenge comes your way.

Warm your core up with the core-empowering stretches for approximately thirty seconds, then hold a static stretch at the end ranges for another thirty seconds for a total duration of at least sixty seconds. The American College of Sports Medicine recommends doing stretches for a minimum of one minute. These cyclical movements will increase your core awareness and develop the foundation for a powerful and resilient core, reducing your risk of injury. These, of course, are simply recommendations and not dogma. Listen to your own body and choose what feels good for you. Remember to stop any movement that causes you to feel pain, or if you cannot maintain proper alignment and technique during a movement.

One mechanism you should consider when performing these exercises is the stretch reflex, a signal transmitted from sensory receptors inside your muscles to the central nervous system that detects abrupt and uncontrolled changes in muscle length. Activating the stretch reflex resists the change in length by causing the muscle to contract, protecting you from unwanted injuries. This is your body's way of saying "that's too far!" To avoid the protective contraction of a stretch reflex that will resist lengthening, perform the stretches slowly, actively, and with precision, controlled awareness, and muscular engagement. You should not try to push the stretches to the point of pain or significant discomfort. You will gradually increase your range of motion and core control faster and more safely by moving slowly, breathing deeply, and focusing your awareness on your body and movements.

Progress slowly and gradually so your muscles can get used to longer stretches and ultimately achieve greater flexibility by combining your breath with your movement. Never hold or force your breath. Instead, follow its natural rhythm, and pair your inhalations with positions that open or expand your chest while you stretch out taller and raise your arms overhead. Conversely, your body naturally wants to exhale when you fold inward or twist. The Core BASE provides suggestions for coordinating inhalation and exhalations with movement. As you practice and connect with your core, you will learn to explore your own breath with these core-empowering dynamic stretches to become long and strong. Blessed are the flexible, for they will not be bent out of shape!

Core-Empowering Stretches

"Nothing happens until something moves."
—Albert Einstein

Core Stretch #1: Awaken and Grow

Awaken and grow your core by combining diaphragmatic breathing with axial extension, or lengthening your spine along its axis. This full body stretch relieves compression and muscle tension by increasing the space between your vertebrae (the bones of your spine) to counteract the effects of gravity. Height loss is an age-related phenomenon caused by changes in muscles, bones, and joints. On average, men lose an inch of height between ages thirty and seventy, while women lose an average of two inches within the same period.

The goal is to create space in your core by lengthening your body into maximum vertical alignment. Lie on your back with a neutral head and neck position (not tilted up or down), with your arms at your sides, palms facing up, smiling with your collarbones, and spreading your wings to open your ribcage. Perform axial extension by stretching your body in both directions (up with the top of your head, and down with your feet). Imagine yourself growing taller as you lengthen your spine on inhalation, taking slow, deep breaths.

As you exhale, draw in your core muscles by "toning" your belly and lifting your core floor while maintaining the integrity of your spinal curves to optimally engage your inner core muscles. Conversely, posterior tilting, or "flexing" of the pelvis, which is still erroneously advocated in many "core stability" programs, flattens the lower back and takes the spine away from its optimal neutral position, rendering the inner core muscles ineffective. As you tone your belly, flex your feet up with your toes pointing toward your nose as you exhale, while lengthening your body from your heels to your head. Next, raise your arms up in a "Y" position as you inhale and stretch up through your fingers and down through your toes, then lower your arms back to your sides while you tone your belly again upon exhalation.

Core Stretch #2: Core Butterfly

Once you have awakened and lengthened your core in the longitudinal plane (from top to bottom), we can move on to the Core Butterfly exercise to focus more on the expansion of your core cylinder in the transverse plane (front to back, and side to side). This dynamic exercise promotes the stretching of your chest, abdomen, and pelvic floor, increases lung expansion, and elicits inner core activation.

Begin the Core Butterfly on your back in a hook lying position, with your knees comfortably bent, feet together on the ground, and arms at your sides. Inhale as you slowly slide your arms up to a "Y" position with your elbows straight, and then allow your knees to slowly drop out to the sides into a butterfly shape. Depending upon your own flexibility, your knees might touch the floor, or may just hang in a relaxed position.

At first, it can be helpful to move your arms and legs into position sequentially. Inhale to focus on expanding your upper chest and ribs as your breath starts to come in, then shift focus to the lower part of your cylinder as your legs open. As you exhale, bring your arms and legs back to the original position as you tone your core, squeeze your legs together, and engage all of your inner core muscles, including your pelvic floor. For added stretch, you can place blocks or pillows under your trunk.

Core Stretch #3: Trunk Twist

After the core cylinder has been dynamically stretched from top to bottom, side to side, and front to back, the next step is to stretch by rotating along the transverse plane with a Trunk Twist. A rotational stretch lengthens, relaxes, and realigns your core while hydrating your spinal discs and gently stretching the joints in your spine to release natural endorphins and lubrication.

Begin this dynamic stretch on your back, with your inner core toned and arms on the floor in a "Y" position, just like the Core Butterfly. Raise your feet off the ground and bring your knees toward your chest until your hips and knees form a 90-degree angle. Inhale as you slowly rotate your legs to one side, and exhale as you bring them back up. Repeat on the other side and progressively increase the excursion, or how far your legs go, with each repetition.

If this stretch feels too aggressive you can modify it by starting with the soles of your feet on the ground, making small motions with your knees until you gradually progress to larger excursions toward the ground. To advance this exercise, lift your legs off the ground to a position of 90 degrees at your hips and knees, and cross your bottom leg over your top leg at the end of the excursion for added stretch.

Core Stretch #4: Dynamic Cat

The Dynamic Cat stretches the core in all of the aforementioned planes of motion. This stretch brings the trunk into extension (or an arched position), flexion (rounded position), and lateral flexion (side-bending). Start by positioning yourself in a quadruped position (on your hands and knees, with hands directly under your shoulders, and knees directly under your hips). Lengthen your entire spine in its natural neutral alignment by imagining yourself as a turtle coming out of its shell and elongating its neck.

Imagine a string pulling your navel toward the ground by making a "C" shape of your trunk, with the open part of the "C" facing toward the sky. As your belly drops, open your chest by smiling with your collarbones and pulling your shoulder blades back and down. Exaggerate the curve in your back by looking up to the sky, lengthening your neck, and lifting your tailbone by sticking out your butt. Link your breath to this movement by inhaling through your nose as your belly drops and your core cylinder expands. Be sure to isolate the movement to your trunk, keeping your arms straight and thighs perpendicular to the ground.

Now exhale as you round your back upwards like an angry cat, with the open part of the "C" now facing the ground. Tone your core as you imagine the string now pulling your navel to the heavens, and another string pulling your head to your tailbone. As you exhale, tuck your tailbone, arch your back, and drop your head so that your gaze comes toward your navel. Let your cat roar as you exhale forcefully through your mouth and stick your tongue out to open and relax your jaw and throat.

Finally, incorporate side flexion by moving your hips in a circular motion to provide additional stretch to the trunk, hips, and pelvic floor. Listen to your body as you customize this stretch to meet your own needs, gradually incorporating multi-directional movements. If the quadruped position is problematic due to extremity issues (such as knee or shoulder pain), these same dynamic stretches may be performed from standing or sitting positions.

Core Stretch #5: Dynamic Dog

To transition from the Dynamic Cat to the Dynamic Dog starting position, push up from your hands and knees by lifting your knees away from the floor and pushing your hips toward the sky. Make sure your arms and legs are straight but not locked, heels stretched down toward the ground, butt lifted toward the sky, spine in its natural neutral alignment, and your head and neck relaxed.

This inverted position, with your heart above your head, encourages circulation to nourish your core and your entire body. It also targets your hamstring muscles, which influence pelvic positioning for optimal inner core muscle activation and spinal health. Inhale as you gently lower to a plank position by shifting your weight forward and slowly moving your hips down to form a straight line with your trunk and legs, keeping your collarbones "smiling".

Continue your inhalation as you lower your hips toward the ground with your arms still extended, allowing your lower back to sag into a backbend for maximal expansion of your core cylinder. Exhale as you tone your core and push back up to the starting position. The Dynamic Dog may be modified, if necessary, by performing the same movement with your arms on a stable chair or low counter until sufficient core flexibility and strength are established.

Core Stretch #6: Heart Opener

Chances are, your daily activities require you to be hunched over for the majority of your day, causing a forward rolled posture that shortens your chest and abdominal muscles while weakening your inner core muscles. The Heart Opener stretches these tight muscles and improves your posture for optimal core muscle functioning.

Begin this stretch by standing tall with your feet hip-width apart, each of your ten toes connected with the Earth, and one arm placed behind your lower back. Raise the other arm behind your head, reaching for the first arm. If possible, clasp the fingers of each hand together, or modify with a towel, strap, or belt. Inhale as you reach and open your heart, smile with your collarbones, then exhale as you release and relax. Repeat with opposite hands.

Next, clasp your hands behind your hips (or modify by holding on to a towel or strap), push your chest forward as you inhale, and pull your shoulders down and away from your ears. Exhale as you release and tone your core.

Core Stretch #7: Tree in the Wind

The Tree in the Wind dynamic stretch brings us full circle, reinforcing the initial stretch for axial extension by lengthening the entire body from toes to fingertips in a standing position, thus challenging your core to resist the effects of gravity.

Stand with your feet hip-width apart and reach your arms toward the sky in a "Y" position. Inhale as you tilt your trunk and arms to one side, reaching through your fingertips while simultaneously pushing through the opposite foot into the ground and making sure not to lean forward or backward. Exhale as you return to the original stance. Repeat on the other side, again making sure to sync your breath with your motion for optimal core activation.

Next, with your arms still overhead, stretch your head and trunk backward as you slowly arch your back. This stretch can be modified by simply standing in front of a counter and gently moving your hips forward. Always listen to your body, and never force any motions that don't feel right.

Table 1. The Core-Empowering Stretches:

This table illustrates the phases of the seven core-stretching exercises. These slow dynamic movements combined with diaphragmatic breathing, prepare the core for sustained stretches at end range for optimal core flexibility. Warm your core up with these dynamic stretches for approximately thirty seconds of fluid movement through all three phases, then hold a static sustained stretch at the end ranges for another thirty seconds, for a total duration of at least sixty seconds.

Table 1. The Core Stretching 7

Dynamic Core Stretch	Phase 1	Phase 2	Phase 3
Awaken & Grow			
Core Butterfly			
Trunk Twist			
Dynamic Cat			
Dynamic Dog			
Heart Opener			
Tree in the Wind			

Seeds for Thought

- Have you tried lengthening your exhalations to calm your nervous system during a stressful situation?
- During which of your daily activities did you practice toning your core?
- Did tuning in to the natural engagement of your inner core muscles with your breath help improve and support your posture?
- Which core-empowering stretches were your favorites?
- How did you feel before and after performing them?

CHAPTER 10

Awareness

"Self-awareness is the most important thing towards being
a champion."
—Billie Jean King

Once you have established the foundation of deep, diaphragmatic breathing to align and awaken your inner core squad in the Breathing Phase of the Core BASE Guide, the Awareness Phase will develop your mind-core connection with meditation, empowering mantras, and scientifically-based muscle activation exercises to strengthen your whole team of local and global core muscles. Activation and strength of your core muscles is necessary for balance, control, and coordination of your trunk muscles as the powerhouse of your body.

Over five hundred years ago, Leonardo da Vinci first observed the mysterious, universal growth pattern in the size of a tree's trunk and its branches. Da Vinci wrote, "All the branches of a tree at every stage of its height, when put together, are equal in thickness to the trunk." So, if a tree's branches are folded upward and squeezed together, the tree would look like one big trunk, with the same thickness from top to bottom. This amazing structural phenomenon is related to a tree's ability to withstand stress, much like the ability of the human body, as stability and resilience of all segments are directly related to stability of the trunk.

Da Vinci's astute observation correlated the size of the trunk with stability of the body. Stability of the human body is dependent not just upon size and strength of the trunk, but also the ability to activate the trunk muscles for coordinated movement. In his depictions of the spine, Da Vinci recognized how important it was for the inner core muscles to work together for functional movement, "like the side-riggings of a mast of a ship." Core muscle strength and muscle activation are interrelated and equally important for optimal functioning of your body, but they are not the same thing. Think of a muscle-bound body builder who can bench press 400 pounds, but lacks the functional muscle activation to wrestle an MMA fighter half his size. The fighter has trained his mind and muscles to activate his body with explosive and resilient strength and agility to meet the variable physical demands of real-world circumstances.

Strength is your muscle's ability to produce force: the stronger your muscle, the more force it can produce. This is necessary for moving loads, such as when you are lifting a suitcase. Strength is also important when you are resisting forces that are applied to your body, like when you maintain your stance through the sudden starts and stops of the subway, hit a curb on your bicycle, or try to keep your balance when your dog jumps off of your surfboard. Your muscles' ability to switch on and function is known as muscle activation. Muscle activation is dependent upon a solid mind-muscle connection. A stronger connection between your mind and muscles will make the muscles more active, which means your brain will have an easier time recruiting a particular muscle to meet functional demands. This is what gives you agility, or the ability to make quick and reflexive postural adjustments in direction and speed.

The mind-core connection ensures that you are using the right muscles at the right time to move the way you intend to. This concept is important, because in order to move efficiently and safely, you need the appropriate muscles to work. The saying, "All roads lead to Rome" also applies to movement. There are many ways that you can perform a particular movement, but some ways are safer and more efficient than others.

For example, let's look at a simple shoulder movement, like reaching to grab a carton of milk from your fridge. You have many muscles within the shoulder complex that can assist with this movement for stability and movement of the arm. When some muscles are weak or in pain, they may not "turn on" at the right time or with the right intensity for fluid, pain-free movement. As a result, other muscles may become overactive in order to compensate, which may further complicate biomechanics.

Muscle activation is good, but over-activation is not necessarily a good thing, as it may pull your mechanics out of balance. Take a look at your shoulders in a mirror when you raise your arms and see if you notice a difference between the left and right sides. If you notice a difference, it may be due to muscle activation. With faulty biomechanics, you are more likely to have pain and injury.

All movements of the body are unique, and the contribution needed from each of your core muscles varies with each task, requiring more or less activation to fine tune your movement. Muscles can become too active, but they can also become inactive when they should be firing to support your movements. The reason certain muscles become overactive and others underactive is often due to your habits, sustained poor posture, and repetitive movements that cause muscles to become imbalanced.

Scientific evidence supports core stabilization exercises as the foundation for building greater core awareness by teaching your mind to activate and strengthen the muscles of your abdomen, back, inner core, and glutes. These exercises incorporate arm and leg movements synergistically with the conscious awareness of your inner core, specifically your diaphragm, transversus abdominis, pelvic floor, and multifidus muscles in rhythm with the power of your breath. The inner core toner starts the core engine, while the core awareness exercises get the core engine firing on all cylinders. These exercises add forces through your trunk and limbs to functionally reinforce the optimal pattern of proximal stability for distal mobility.

Brace Yourself for Whatever Comes Your Way

"The key to growth is the introduction of higher dimensions of consciousness into our awareness."
—Lao Tzu

You must learn to tune your core tone to match the activity that you are performing, like when you are sitting, standing, walking, squatting, or lifting throughout your day, all of which require your core muscles to work together. Whenever you are performing any type of activity, like standing up from a chair, climbing stairs, or leaning over your sink, global muscle activity kicks in to reinforce your anatomical girdle of the inner core muscles. For example, picking up a pencil from the ground will require much less global core muscle activation than performing a 300-pound deadlift, which would require maximal bracing of all your trunk muscles. To get an idea of how you can maximally brace your core, imagine protecting yourself from a punch to your belly.

Core stability is not just strength or stiffness; it is dynamic balance and coordination of your muscular control. The balance and coordinated action of your core muscles is what develops your resiliency, just like the tree that bends but doesn't break from the forces of the wind. The full excursion of your inner core in expanding and activating your core is important for healthy functioning. A self-conscious girl who has forced herself to suck in her belly, as well as a body builder with strong, tight abs, are both vulnerable to injuring their "armadillo shell," which has forgotten how to soften and respond on demand.

Throughout all of our movements, we are always creating some level of core bracing, but trying to brace your core at 100 percent all the time will put constant pressure up against your diaphragm and down against your core floor. Over time, this constant pressure will limit the range of movement in your core muscles, create stiffness and weakness, and affect your breathing, core health, and overall functioning. It is equally important to both contract and release all of your core muscles, as a soft and relaxed core fosters openness and relaxation, and is key for letting go and melting the armor of your core and heart.

It's critical that you do these exercises often so you update your software for optimal movement. Only through repetition, awareness, proper breathing, and proper movement will you be able to create the core software and hardware needed to maintain this pattern of movement throughout every motion you make in life, which is the ultimate goal of this program. The dynamic multi-joint training exercises you'll learn here are paramount for injury prevention, and mimic core muscle activation that is similar to the activation patterns in daily activities and sports.

Core-Empowering Meditation to Unite Mind-Body-Spirit

"When meditation is mastered, the mind is unwavering, like the
flame of a candle in a windless place."
—Veda Vyasa

Meditation is a vital component of the Awareness Phase of the BASE Guide, and also important for establishing the mind-core connection. You possess an ocean of unconscious mind-core power, so let's dive in!

Find a comfortable position and allow your body to relax. Begin by assuming a strong and open posture based on your flexibility and comfort level. You can try sitting cross-legged, kneeling, sitting, standing, or even floating on a paddleboard. Liberate your mind from the grip of your thoughts. Put aside all of your connections and imagine there is no one else in the world for this moment.

Bring attention to the position of your core and maintain the natural curve of your spine without straining. Your back should be strong and stable, with your front relaxed and open to encourage your breath, blood, and energy to circulate freely throughout your body. Give your body permission to let go of tension, allowing your muscles to soften. Bring the focus of your awareness to your breath.

Breathe deeply and slowly, first into your belly, then ribs, and chest, and reverse the flow with a slow exhale from yor belly, then ribs, and chest. Place your hands on your abdomen and feel your belly rise and fall. Breathe in joy, breathe out tension. Breathe in harmony, breathe out discord. Breathe in healing, breathe out disease. Inhale calm, exhale stress. Next, place your hands on your lower ribs and feel them expand and recede with each breath in and out, like the waves of the sea.

Draw your attention to your trunk muscles as you begin the inner core toner exercise and coordinate activation with your diaphragmatic breathing. Do not allow your mind to wander. Establish your foundation of core stability as you connect your mind with your inner core, focusing on toning your core (contracting) with your exhalations and melting (relaxing) with your inhalations. It's very important that you learn to relax well and let go of tension in your mind and body, softening your face, jaw, neck, shoulders, core, and legs. Training your core is just as much about learning to relax your muscles as it is learning to contract them. Remember, core control is the goal, which means you must be able to generate the right amount of strength at the right time, while also being able to relax completely when your muscles don't need to be activated.

Draw a mental image of all the segments of your body. Now, channel the energy from your core to each of those body parts individually, beginning with your feet. Tone your core as you exhale and tighten your muscles. As you inhale, relax your core and the individual muscle groups that you are focusing on in that moment. Begin by contracting your calves and the bottoms of your feet as you flex your toes away from your nose. As you inhale, relax your core and feet. Slowly work your way through the muscles of your body: the tops of your feet, the front of your hips and thighs, the back of your thighs and glutes, and your fingers, hands, and arms. Tighten each muscle group in rhythm with your core contractions and breathing.

Once you achieve harmony in this rhythm of mind-core awareness, detach your mind as the controller. Become an objective observer, or a nonreactive monitor of your body, by simply perceiving and developing awareness without judgment. Observe the input from all of your senses, especially your sixth sense of proprioception. With your mind in this monitoring state, you will make new brain connections that will deepen your awareness of your breath, posture, and core function.

Meditation empowers your body and mind to flow together. Connecting your body's energy to universal energy will ground you and bring you a sense of peace, stability, and heightened core awareness. The core is a place of great sensation with tremendous emotion and energy, because there are more nerve cells in your belly than in your entire peripheral nervous system. Meditation is a powerful tool for harnessing this vast resource of energy and information that is already inside you. All you need to do is tap into it with your awareness and train your mind to pay attention to what's within you, instead of everything that's outside you.

Core-Empowering Mantras to Replenish Your Inner Core Garden

"The energy of the mind is the essence of life."
—Aristotle

For thousands of years, many spiritual traditions have used mantras as a strategy for calming and focusing the mind. This ancient practice has been validated by brain imaging as beneficial for your health. Repeating a word or group of words exerts a wide array of emotional and cognitive effects, and can help to calm mental chatter while also facilitating deep absorption and transcendence to mystical states.

In Eastern traditions, "mantra" is a word of Sanskrit origin from the words "mana," which means "mind," and "tra," which means "tool." A mantra is an instrument of thought that transports or elevates your mind to a deeper awareness and spirituality. In Western culture, the term "mantra" is synonymous with an affirmation. A mantra is repeated silently, or whispered over and over to transcend the activity of the mind. It is simply a strategy that helps you access heightened levels of awareness.

Repeating mantras or positive affirmations, coordinated with the rhythm of your breath, will help you replace negative thought patterns with positive ones to build your mental, emotional, and spiritual muscles. For thousands of years, Buddhists, Hindus, Taoists, Native Americans, and many other cultures all over the world have coordinated spoken, sung, or mentally repeated phrases with exhalation, followed by a pause for slow inhalation.

Mantras maintain and replenish the health of your inner garden and awaken your appreciation for the beauty and wonder of life that is always around you. A mantra is the seed which must be nurtured to bear the fruit of your intention. Neuroscientists are now recognizing the benefits of mantras in alleviating negative emotions, fostering positive ones, calming your nervous system, and increasing awareness and focus for your exercises, your goals, and your life.

One of the goals of developing this awareness is to feel more present and peaceful. The benefits of this more calm, aware state will flow into every other aspect of your life. Repeating these affirmations silently or aloud during exercise cultivates mind-core focus to help you achieve your goals. The core exercises are the postures of the body, whereas the mantras are postures of the mind and spirit. Empowering mantras or affirmations improve your self-confidence, awareness, and positive thinking. As you repeat these mantras with self-love and faith, feel yourself expand and grow into an even more powerful and magnificent being.

Developing the perception of diaphragmatic breathing, trunk stretching, and core activation with these core-empowering mantras allows you to proceed with more challenging stabilization exercises that evoke high activity of the core musculature. Empowering mantras provide a strong foundation for more focused mind, body, and spirit awareness to guide you in your progression through the exercises of the Core BASE Guide. You will get the most benefits out of this program (and any other fitness program) when you train your mind as well as your body.

Core Mantras

I am in control.
I choose positivity.
I will challenge my core.
I find strength in adversity.
I have potential for greatness.
I will listen to my body.
I believe in my core.

Cultivating Body Awareness

"The mind's first step to self-awareness must be through the body."
—George Sheehan

"No pain, no gain" is a catchphrase popularized by Jane Fonda's aerobics videos from the 1980s. This exercise motto promises rewards for the price of pain. This concept dates back to Benjamin Franklin ("no gain without pain") and Nietzsche ("what does not kill me makes me stronger"). There is no doubt that hard work and struggle build both psychological and physical strength and resilience, but this motto has regrettably been misconstrued and has caused a vast amount of unfortunate injuries, as I have witnessed over my career. Exercising while in pain is a common mistake, and it is time to debunk this erroneous myth. The key word that has been misconstrued is "pain," as pain is complex, multi-faceted, and means different things to different people.

Cultivating body awareness will help you understand the difference between detrimental pain and beneficial pain (really more accurately described as "discomfort") during exercise. This awareness will help you avoid a serious or long-term injury on your path to peak core fitness. Pay attention to the warning cues that your body provides to maintain a safe and effective training routine. It is important that you learn to distinguish what your body's sensations are telling you. If you are experiencing pain, stop for a moment and try to discern what type of pain you are feeling.

Learning to distinguish the difference between pain and discomfort when training can be tricky, as everyone has a unique perception and threshold for pain. Detrimental pain is your body's warning signal, often localized deep in your joints or bones, and alerts you to a potential problem. It tends to come on suddenly, and is sharp, shooting, aching, or irritating. It quickly catches your attention precisely because you are meant to listen and act on any such perceptions. Exercise should not cause this type of pain, and if it does, you should back off or stop the activity until the pain subsides. Any pain felt at the start of an exercise should be a warning sign that something is wrong. A severe or sharp pain during a workout indicates that something in your body is stressed, inflamed, damaged, or sensitive. Do not push through it. It is risky behavior to ignore this type of pain by working or pushing through the pain. The odds of developing a serious or chronic injury (such as tendonitis, bursitis, or stress fractures) increase as you exercise with pain.

Listen to your body and look for red flags that indicate injury, such as swelling and bruising. Injuries are usually, though not always, accompanied by sounds and sensations. You may hear or feel a popping or snapping sound or sensation if you've torn a muscle or ligament, or a cracking sound if you injure a joint. However, your joints often make noises that do not signal injury. These sounds are called "crepitus," which refers to harmless grinding, creaking, crunching, and/or popping (such as when you crack your knuckles) without the presence of pain. Swelling and redness are two major signs of inflammation, a key indicator that your body is trying to heal something. If you're injured, you'll most likely experience swelling in a localized area, which may be tender to the touch.

Discomfort, on the other hand, is often a normal part of exercise training and can be an indication that your workouts are challenging you to improve your strength and endurance. Muscle fatigue is a sensation in the muscles that is experienced as a burning feeling. A true muscle burn will be perceived as an increase in heat, and your muscles will start to feel heavy. Once you cannot complete a movement without any compensation, then you know your muscles are fatigued, and you should rest before attempting that activity again. People who exercise regularly recognize this feeling of burning or fatigue in their muscles when they push a little harder out of their comfort zone.

Understanding what's happening inside your body promotes awareness. When you push a muscle to work beyond its ability to use oxygen delivered in the blood, you're creating lactic acid. This production of lactic acid is what gives you that burning sensation, which actually plays a role in creating more blood flow to the muscles so that you gain more strength and endurance. Experienced exercisers strive to "feel the burn," knowing that this is a good fatigue, not detrimental pain, and important for gains in training.

Discomfort in your muscles, or delayed onset muscle soreness (DOMS), usually begins the day after exercise and may linger for up to three days after training, particularly after an intense session. This sort of discomfort, while not pleasant, is a normal response to using muscles that are unaccustomed to a particular activity. With any challenging training regiment, dull, achy soreness in your muscles is normal for up to three days. It's your body's way of letting you know you have pushed yourself and challenged your muscles. Although not yet completely understood by scientists, DOMS is the feeling you get when your muscle fibers microscopically tear during training and then repair during rest and recovery.

Deliberately tearing your muscles may seem counterintuitive, but the process of rebuilding these micro-tears is necessary for building muscle mass, or hypertrophy. You have to break down to build stronger, more powerful, and more resilient muscles. Generalized swelling after a workout is due to a build-up of fluids, including water and blood, as well as nutrients and other particles your body sends to help repair the muscles. If you do experience DOMS swelling, it will usually appear over a large area, usually the entire muscle that is sore, unlike the localized swelling from an injury. Delayed muscle soreness is only felt in the muscles, not the joints or tendons.

Even the most fit people can get muscle soreness if they do something new or add duration or intensity to their exercise. When you feel DOMS, this indicates that your body needs time to heal and recover before your next workout. Pushing yourself to train again while you are in a DOMS state can lead to injury. This can occur because your joints and muscles may be less able to absorb impact, forcing potentially injurious compensations for the fatigued muscle. Additionally, muscle soreness changes your perceived intensity, meaning that you could push your muscles too much and lead to overuse injuries. If your body does not get the required rest time needed for recovery, it may have counterproductive effects that lead to too much stress and can cause muscle strains, as the muscle may not have its full shock attenuation properties, may limit range of motion, or can be temporarily weaker while recovering.

Although it is important to rest after strenuous exercise, remaining completely sedentary actually makes DOMS worse. Although it's tempting to hit the couch when you are sore, you can speed up your recovery time with low- to moderate- intensity movement. The best way to find relief is to engage in gentle activity that gets your blood flowing. Strategies to decrease DOMS for quicker recovery include applying ice, massaging, and engaging in light cardiovascular exercise, such as walking, jogging, swimming, cycling, rowing, or biking.

It's important to note that these same principles do not apply to the heart. Cardiovascular muscle gains are different than the rest of your body's muscles; the heart can get stronger and more efficient at less than maximum fatigue. If your heart is beating at a moderately faster rate, you will not feel pain, yet your heart muscle will still benefit. If you begin to experience pain in your chest, or feel lightheaded or dizzy while exercising, slow down, especially if you are over the age of thirty-five. Cardiovascular disease is the leading cause of death among people thirty-five and older. Check with your doctor about any symptoms of pressure or tightness under your breastbone. If you're younger than thirty-five and feel chest pain, it's unlikely to be a heart problem, but it's still a good idea to stop the activity and consult your doctor.

For safe exercise progression, only increase your training intensity or duration as long as you are pain-free and have full range of motion without joint soreness. Do not increase exercise intensity more than 5 to 10 percent per week. This general guideline will keep your training in line with your body's ability to progress. Get in tune with your body as it adapts to change; exercise should not cause pain. Sharp, deep, or lasting pain needs to be respected! If exercise does cause pain, you are either doing it incorrectly, have not fully recovered from an injury, or may be on your way to developing a chronic injury. Be mindful of the subtle—and not-so-subtle—warning signs your body provides and adjust your exercise accordingly to avoid pain and get great results. Developing your own body awareness wisdom comes with time and experience. Don't consider a lighter workout a defeat, but a steppingstone on your journey to core empowerment!

Core Awareness Exercise

"Awareness is like the sun. When it shines on things, they are
transformed."
—Thich Nhat Hanh

Are you ready for your core "aha" moment? It's time to feel
your core in action! The core awareness exercises should always be
preceded by a few deep diaphragmatic breaths and inner core toners
as you visualize the task ahead. Begin each exercise as you exhale and
contract your inner core to prepare your body for the upcoming load.
Try to sustain this tension deep inside while your global muscles start
chiming in. This is when you begin to experience the full symphony of
all the members of your core orchestra performing together!

Core Awareness Exercise #1: Bug

The Bug is an excellent preliminary exercise for promoting
stabilization of the core muscles, as well as building motor skills and
coordination. The Bug is performed on your back in the hook lying
position, and begins with the conscious awareness of your inner core as
you lift your pelvic floor toward your spine while tightening your inner
core muscles. Be sure to maintain the integrity of your natural spinal
curves to optimally engage your core muscles.

Practice this maneuver by drawing in your abdominal muscles, as
if tightening a corset around your waist. Release your core and repeat,
tightening your core with each exhalation. Once you've established
conscious awareness of your inner core, exhale as you contract your
inner core muscles prior to movement. Raise your arms overhead,
alternating your left and right arms and synchronizing your movements
with the power of your breath. Feel your global muscles kicking in.
Progress to alternately lifting your legs to a position of 90 degrees at
your hips and knees.

Try an advanced version of the Bug by synchronizing opposite
arm and leg movements. While lowering your right arm and left leg,
raise your left arm and right leg. Alternate your arm and leg motion
in a rhythmic, steady march, in sync with your breathing. To further
challenge your core, try adding multi-directional limb movements, like

a ladybug stuck on its back. Flail your limbs at varying speeds or add resistance bands for increased core muscle activation.

Core Awareness Exercise #2: Bridge

The Bridge is an excellent exercise for progressing core activation while targeting your core and glutes. Lie on your back with your knees comfortably bent and feet on the ground. Experiment with different placements of your feet to find the position that feels best for your body.

Slowly take a deep breath in; then, as you exhale, lift your pelvic floor, tone your inner core, clench your glutes, and press your feet into the ground while you lift your trunk up from the lowest vertebra to the highest, forming a straight, long, strong line from your shoulders to your knees. Be sure not to lift your hips higher than a straight line, as this may put excessive strain on your lower back.

In the bridge position, ensure your trunk is toned, and lengthen through the front of your hips. Then, slowly lower down one vertebra at a time from the neck to the tailbone. If this is too challenging, simply begin with clenching your glutes and initiate lifting your hips. For progression of the bridge, increase the intensity by squeezing a ball or block between your knees to promote more core floor activation, or by adding resistance bands around your thighs. Additional variations include lifting each leg alternately off the ground or lifting your heels.

Core Awareness Exercise #3: Bird Dog

The Bird Dog exercise builds the core activation established in the Bug and Bridge to further challenge your core musculature. The quadruped position (on your hands and knees) reinforces proper spinal alignment and postural control. This exercise challenges your core by raising your center of gravity and teaches the discipline of coordinated arm and leg motion with a stable trunk.

Inhale slowly and deeply while maintaining a neutral spine with its natural curves. Exhale as you lift your pelvic floor. Tone your trunk and raise your arm and opposite leg straight out in one line with your trunk, making sure not to sway or twist your pelvis. Inhale as you relax and return to the original position, and exhale as you switch arms and legs. The goal of this exercise is to resist the forces that destabilize your spine and cause you to lose balance. If you find it too challenging, this exercise may be modified by leaning over a chair, table, or countertop, or quadruped with isolated arm or leg motions until core control is sufficient to combine alternate motions. You can also modify by placing a pillow or cushion under your belly.

If you want to challenge yourself more, add arm and leg motions to further ramp up the global core muscle activation. Resistance bands may also be used with your arm or leg motions. You may also shift your weight forward through your weight-bearing arm, floating the weightbearing knee off the ground to provide additional destabilizing forces, which increases your core muscle recruitment.

Core Awareness Exercise #4: Plank

The plank exercise has been extensively researched and found to promote high core muscle activation. This exercise involves positioning your body face-down with your forearms and toes on the ground. With your elbows directly under your shoulders and your fingers facing forward, prop your body up off the ground. Your head should remain in a neutral alignment, with your gaze toward the floor to avoid neck strain.

As you exhale, draw your core floor up toward your spine to tone your belly and engage the core muscles. Focus on keeping your trunk rigid in a neutral spine position, or a straight line from head to toe, with no sagging or arching. Arching of the back indicates inadequate inner core muscle activation, while sagging hips indicate fatigue, which means it's time to end the plank. To modify the plank, begin by planking on your knees, or perform an incline plank by resting your forearms on a high table or counter.

To advance the plank, progress to weight-bearing through the hands instead of forearms (you should be in push-up position), and by incorporating shoulder taps to the opposite shoulder to increase core activity and stabilize while balancing on one arm. For further core challenge, lift one leg at a time to further promote increased activation of the global core musculature.

Core Awareness Exercise #5: Side Plank

The side plank further increases awareness of the core and elicits high back and side trunk muscle activation, while kicking in greater coordination of the deep abdominals. To perform the side plank, lie on your side with your legs fully extended and stacked on top of each other. Upon exhalation, lift your core floor and tone your belly to engage your inner core, and use your elbow and your forearm to prop your body up in a straight line from your head to your toes.

Keep your core tight and your neck in line with your body. Avoid raising or dropping your head. Be aware of your hip position, as sagging or dropping indicates fatigue, at which point the exercise should be stopped. Repeat on the other side. If you find this exercise too challenging, it can be modified by performing the side plank on a bent knee, or even a chair or high counter, which allows beginners to progressively adapt to the core demands of this challenging exercise. Advance your core awareness by progressing to weight-bearing through your hand instead of your forearm.

For a dynamic progression, try slowly lifting your top arm and/or leg toward the sky like a starfish, then back to the starting position while maintaining alignment of the limbs and trunk in one plane. To challenge the core even further, try a "Turkish get up," which is a transition from lying on your side to a standing position while extending your upper arm toward the sky (like in the starfish side plank) throughout the entire exercise. This advanced functional movement first involves pushing through the lower leg and elbow from your side to a seated position. From the seated position, push through your hand, lift your hips, and slide your lower leg underneath your body, stepping back and settling onto your knee before pushing up through your legs from the half-kneeling position to stand.

Core Awareness Exercise #6: Squat

The squat, a phenomenal standing core activator, is known as the "king" of core exercises because it is a fundamental movement pattern we learn as babies while trying to stabilize our center of gravity for our first steps. In this core awareness exercise, the hips are lowered from an upright standing position, which fires up your trunk muscles and posterior chain. The movement pattern of this seat of power is required for sitting, lifting, and sports, and is a staple exercise in injury prevention and performance enhancement training programs.

To perform this exercise, stand as tall as possible with your feet hip-width apart, and your arms in front of you to maintain your balance. Keeping your back in its natural alignment, inhale as you drop your hips and sit back into an imaginary chair as you tilt your trunk forward, until your thighs are parallel to the floor. Make sure to keep your knees behind your toes. Pause in this athletic position, with your weight resting slightly more on your heels to engage your core, while your trunk is elongated forward and up. As you exhale, lift your core floor and tone your trunk as you drive through your heels to lift back to the starting position. If you have significant core weakness, the exercise may be initiated by standing with your back against the wall, or squatting to a high chair until more core control is developed. The core musculature, particularly the pelvic floor, is activated while descending into the squat position, and contracted or lifted when coming up.

To further challenge your core, try variations of this exercise, such as squatting with a resistance band around your thighs, or side-stepping in the squatting position with the band. Hip muscle activity may be augmented during resisted side-stepping in multiple directions, or while maintaining the athletic squat with different band positions. Compared with placing the band around your ankles, placing the band around your feet for resisted side-stepping elicits more activity in the gluteal muscles that provide proximal stability for your body's chain. Further challenge your core by adding hand weights to your double leg squats, progressing to single leg squats on both sides to balance out asymmetries and decrease your risk of injury throughout your kinetic chain.

Core Awareness Exercise #7: Warrior

The Warrior exercise adds the challenge of balancing on one leg like a bird with spread wings, while controlling your trunk for advanced activation of all your core muscles. Beginners should have the support of a counter or chair nearby for balance if necessary. Inhale as you begin this exercise from a lunge position with your spine in your neutral, natural alignment. Exhale as you lift your core floor, tone your trunk, and shift your weight to your front foot while sweeping your arms back, with your palms facing down. Place your hands on your waist, with your thumbs on your lower ribs and fingertips on the front of your pelvic bones to ensure there is no twisting, while you raise and lower your back leg with control.

The goal is to hinge forward at your hips until your trunk and back leg are parallel to the ground. Flex your back foot and point your toes toward the floor by engaging your core and inner thigh. Broaden your shoulder blades, smile with your collarbones, and lengthen the back of your neck by gazing downward and slightly forward. Engage your standing leg without locking your knee to stabilize and level your hips to the floor. Repeat on the opposite side.

To modify this exercise, simply move through the range of motion where you feel stable and use a block under your hand on the floor for support, or bend your standing leg slightly. For an even easier variation, use a chair or high counter for support. To kick this exercise up a notch, use variations for hand positioning, such as bringing your palms together in a prayer position, moving your lifted leg side to side, or even adding hand weights for an added challenge to the core muscles.

Table 2. Core Awareness Exercises

Table 2 illustrates seven evidence-based core awareness exercises. Each of these core awakeners may be modified or progressed for all core fitness levels.

Begin with one or two sets of 7-12 repetitions of each core awareness exercise. (Rest one minute between sets.) Beginners should hold each repetition for at least five seconds, progressing to a goal of three sets of 7-12 repetitions to develop strength. Work up to holding each posture for thirty seconds after the three sets are completed to develop extra endurance for all your core muscles.

For a more relaxed workout, rest one minute between sets. Or, make your workout more challenging by cycling through the Awareness exercises as a circuit without rest. Never hold your breath! Deep, diaphragmatic breathing should always accompany all exercises. Tighten upon exhalation to start, and then learn to switch up your breathing by tightening on your inhalation, so you can learn to recruit your core muscles throughout the breathing cycle.

Table 2. The Core Awareness 7

Core Awakener	Posture	Modification	Progression
Bug		alternate arms/ alternate legs/ reciprocal limbs	multi-directional limbs/ speed/ resistance band
Bridges		glute sets in hook lying	ball squeeze/ resistance band/ one legged/ heel lift
Bird Dog		leaning over high surface/ quadruped with isolated limb motion	reciprocal limbs/ resistance band/ floating weight bearing knee
Plank		leaning over high surface/ on forearms/ on knees	on hands/ shoulder taps/ alternate leg lift
Side Plank		leaning over high surface/ forearm and bent knee	on hand/ lifting top limbs to sky/ Turkish get up
Squat		wall sits/ shallow squats/ chair squats	resistance band/ side stepping/ hand weights/ single leg
Warrior		support of high surface/ bent standing leg/ block under hand	hands in prayer position/ leg motion/ hand weights

Seeds for Thought

- Have you ever persisted through a workout or activity despite being in pain?

- How did that impact your performance and the way you felt afterward?

- Which core awareness exercises were your favorites? How did you feel before and after performing them?

- Which core awareness exercises did you find most challenging? What was challenging about them?

- Have you felt uplifted by a core-empowering mantra while exercising or simply going about your day? Can you think of creative ways to remember to feed your mind-body-spirit with mantras, such as leaving self-love notes around your house or office, or making them your screensaver?

CHAPTER 11

Stability

"Life is like riding a bicycle. To keep your balance, you must keep moving."
—Albert Einstein

Core empowerment is an evolution, a continuous process of becoming. The Breathing and Awareness Phases provide the foundation for your core health, which is developed through mind-core awareness with the power of your breath. You have learned to pre-activate and engage your trunk muscles. The evidence-based core muscle awareness exercises are important in developing activation and strength of your trunk, yet the roots for true functional stability must be nurtured with functional dynamic tasks that challenge your core and make your neuromuscular system sweat!

The strengthening exercises you have learned thus far work your core muscles in isolation, while keeping the trunk in a neutral position where the majority of the muscles do not change length. For true stability, which is required in many of your real-life daily tasks, you must now incorporate exercises that shorten and lengthen the core muscles to work them in novel ways at different activation levels, and with integrated functional movements of your entire body. For example, your inner core muscles may be only slightly activated while sitting at your desk, whereas they may have to kick into full gear when you lift and lower a heavy package. Other activities require a quick pulse of intense core activation for the split second that you drive a golf ball or hit a baseball.

Your core must be dynamically challenged with external, variable forces to further progress toward empowerment. You have learned to become aware of your center, and now it's time to learn to develop stability for whatever daily task you want to perform. If you have ever tried to whitewater kayak, or even if you haven't had the pleasure, it's easy to imagine what is meant by moving from your center. When you try to maneuver the raging rapids and rocks by simply using your arms to paddle, you will lose your balance and tip over, whereas if you initiate the movement from your core, your stroke will become much more efficient, powerful, and more precise in controlling your trajectory through the current.

Development of core stability is a dynamic process that is unique to each of us, dependent upon your ability to actively control your body and its responses to the forces of your daily activities or even athletic competitions. A dynamically stable core, like a gyroscope, maintains stability with movement while allowing freedom of rotation in all directions. Training for core stability by reinforcing patterns that create greater efficiency in all your movements reduces the risk of injury and prepares you to achieve optimal performance levels in all endeavors.

"There is nothing so stable as change."
—Bob Dylan

In stability training, the goal is to maintain and improve your core neuromuscular control with progressively intense challenges. It is not the strongest that persevere, but the most adaptable, and these exercises will force your body to adapt to many different destabilizing forces. Training facilitates adaptations in your neural superhighway that stabilize all the parts of your body through muscular pre-activation and reactive patterns that protect your body from injurious loading.

Our amazing bodies adapt to whatever we ask of them. The physiological principle of "specificity of training" is important in understanding our muscles' response to training. Essentially, this means that our muscles are creatures of habit, and they get accustomed to the demand we place on them in terms of weight, intensity, duration, speed, and type of movement. Variety is the spice of life, and the essential ingredient in realizing your full potential.

We know that most traumatic injuries occur 40 milliseconds, or 0.04 seconds, after you begin to twist your ankle or knee. That's eight times faster than a blink of your eye! We now also know that lack of core stability is directly linked to injury, and that dynamic training is a key component of injury prevention. Fortunately, you can train your brain, nerves, and muscles to react quickly enough to respond and prevent damage to your body.

When training your core with stability exercises, it's important that you block external distractions and direct your attention to your breath, the natural curve of your spine, and your core tone. Concentrate on a stationary point to become fully present in the moment, and to calm your breath and nervous system. Start by gently looking down the angle of your nose to a point on the floor or the wall.

Do not force a strenuous or intense stare, but rather a soft gaze that rests on one spot. Relax your eyes so that the surrounding visual field comes into subtle awareness. As you become comfortable in the exercise and feel more stable, further challenge your balance by slowly shifting your gaze to the sides and above, moving to the edge of your comfort zone.

Have you ever instinctively closed your eyes to experience all the subtle sounds of a symphony, to fully enjoy the feel of a deep massage, or to savor the taste of melting chocolate on your tongue? When you close your eyes, your gaze turns inward and improves your ability to perceive with your other senses. Your eyes transmit millions of bits of information to your brain every second, and this information plays an important part in your sense of balance and stability. Training without visual cues will provide an extra challenge to your brain and body, helping you further improve your balance and stability while decreasing your risk of injury.

The Dynamic Core Stabilization Phase emphasizes a dual focus of core muscle capacity and control. Stabilizing your core musculature significantly increases core muscular activity during dynamic tasks targeted at improving core proprioception. Prior to each exercise, make sure to take a deep inhalation and incorporate conscious attention to your inner core with every movement. Focus on your inner core muscle tone as you add global core muscle activity to meet the unique functional demands of each exercise. Be sure to tone your core with your back in its natural, neutral alignment, and keep your knees from collapsing into a knock-kneed position.

The Dynamic Core Arsenal provides a plethora of advanced exercises to challenge your core dynamically by using balance exercises, medicine balls, instability devices, plyometric (or hopping) and suspension training (with ropes) activities that teach you to move from your core.

The dynamic variations of the initial core awareness exercises escalate activation of the trunk musculature on your path to core empowerment.

While performing the core stability exercises, focus on your inner core muscles and work on activating the entire perimeter of your trunk, not just the six-pack abs in the front. To help correct a six-pack dominant firing pattern, wrap your hands around your waist periodically and make sure you can feel the tightness of the muscles in your belly, sides, and lower back as you contract your core on all sides (360 degrees). Lightly squeeze or press into your core muscles with your hands to monitor firmness and feel how your local and global muscles work together. This technique will ensure you are not sucking your belly in, but just maintaining tone in an isometric contraction. These core awareness exercises integrate activation of all your core muscles into simple movements as we implement functionally demanding tasks.

During the dynamic stabilization phase, the emphasis is on incorporating fast-paced challenges to the core musculature that involve quickly and repeatedly stretching and contracting your muscles to develop core power, and facilitate adaptations that emphasize control of the entire kinetic chain and are integral to core empowerment. The core dynamic stabilization arsenal will train your core to expect the unexpected, to be prepared to be disturbed, and to meet all the challenges of daily life and sports safely.

Balance

"The balance of power is the scale of peace."
—Thomas Paine

The core is your body's center of balance that controls your positioning during all dynamic tasks. When all the opposing forces acting upon your body are balanced, you are in equilibrium, which is necessary for optimal functioning of your body. Once awareness, activation, and strength of your core muscles are established, the next step is to train your body to move in novel ways that will create a sound, responsive, and enduring sense of balance.

Balance is not something you are born with, nor is it something you find. Rather, it is something you must create and work to maintain through experience and training. In fact, balancing exercises are a key component of all successful injury prevention programs, and should be a priority at any age for the health and well-being of your mind, core, and nervous system.

As you age, your balance deteriorates, unless it is frequently practiced. If you don't use it, you lose it, with "it" referring to both your software (nervous system) and your hardware (musculoskeletal system). Loss of balance impairs the ability to perform daily activities, reduces quality of life, and increases the risk of falling. Each year, one out of every three people over the age of sixty-five will fall, with many of them breaking a bone or sustaining a life-threatening injury. But lack of balance doesn't just cause injuries for the elderly—young people with insufficient balance and poor core control suffer preventable injuries every day while playing sports, working out, or running.

Core balance is dependent upon your ability to integrate sensory elements from your trunk regarding your position in space, as well as your ability to issue commands to the core muscles to make postural adjustments to hold your center of gravity without falling. Your center of gravity (or center of mass) is the exact center around which your body can rotate freely in any direction, and where the weight is equal on all opposing sides.

By challenging your control of your center of gravity, core awareness and core control are developed and brain functioning is improved, all of which are key components for improving reaction time for daily activities, sports, and injury prevention. Improving your core balance will bring grace to all of your movements and power to your punch. If your body is balanced, your mind will be at peace and your spirit will soar!

Core Balance Exercise #1: Y Balance

Imagine a "Y" shape on the floor, or mark one by using tape or drawing lines in the sand. Begin in a standing, upright position in the middle of that "Y" shape (where the stem would meet the two extending arms). Balance on one leg and take turns reaching your other leg, floating your foot slightly above the ground, along each of the three lines. You should feel your core muscles controlling the motion of your stabilizing leg and reaching leg in a fluid motion. Maintain good arch position, and do not allow your heel or big toe to lift off the ground. Repeat on the other side.

Core Balance Exercise #2: Dynamic Warrior

Perform the Warrior exercise as explained in the Awareness Phase of the Core BASE Guide. Once you hinge forward at your hips and your trunk and back leg are parallel to the ground, begin to incorporate some controlled rotation in your trunk. Move your belly button toward your stance leg, and then away to the side. Don't worry if you can't assume the full position parallel to the ground; simply rotate your body over your stance leg to a point where you can hold without losing your balance. Repeat on the other side.

Core Balance Exercise #3: Happy Tree

Begin in an upright, standing position with your arms raised in a "Y" formation. Slowly shift your weight to one leg as you lift the other knee toward your chest as high as possible. Open your lifted leg out to the side by rotating your hip. The sole of your lifted foot should approximate, but not push into, your stance leg. Keep the stance leg straight, but do not lock the knee. Be sure to maintain an upright position with your spine in its natural neutral alignment.

Core Balance Exercise #4: Criss-Cross Crunch

Stand up straight with your legs slightly wider than hip-width apart, and your hands behind your head. Bend your leg and lift your knee as high as you can toward the opposite elbow, while rotating your trunk toward your knee. Avoid locking your stance knee or pulling forward on your neck. Return your trunk and leg to their starting positions as you raise your arms into a "Y" formation. Repeat on the opposite side. For added challenge, try performing the exercise on your toes.

Core Balance Exercise #5: Side Crunch

Stand up straight with your legs slightly wider than hip-width apart, and your hands behind your head. Shift your weight to one side and crunch your trunk to the opposite side as you bring your knee toward your elbow. Lower your leg and return to the start position. Repeat on the opposite side. Keep your spine and neck neutral, your chest up, and your core toned for control to avoid swinging your legs. For added challenge, try performing the exercise on your toes.

Core Balance Exercise #6: Squat Kick

Begin with your legs a little wider than hip-width apart, then drop your hips and sit back into an imaginary chair as you tilt your trunk forward, until your thighs are parallel to the floor. Pause in this athletic position, with your weight resting slightly more on your heels to engage your core, while your trunk is elongated forward and upward. As you return to your standing position, transfer your weight to one leg and kick the other leg out to the side. Repeat this exercise on your other side.

Core Balance Exercise #7: Tree in the Storm

Stand on your toes with your feet slightly wider than hip-width apart, and reach your arms up in a "Y" position. Tilt your trunk and arms to one side, reaching through your fingertips while simultaneously pushing your opposite toes into the ground, making sure to not lean forward or backward. Return to the original stance. Repeat on the other side.

Core Balance Exercises

Table 3 illustrates seven core-empowering balance exercises that challenge your postural control and enhance mind-core connectivity. Progress through these phases slowly, with focus on core control to establish stability. Gradually increase speed and repetitions, working up to three sets of 7-12 repetitions. For added challenge, perform these exercises with weights in your hands.

Table 3. The Core Balance 7

Core Empowering Dynamic Balance Exercises	Phase 1	Phase 2	Phase 3
Y Balance			
Dynamic Warrior			
Happy Tree			
Criss Cross Crunch			
Side Crunch			
Squat Kick			
Tree in the Storm			

Med Balls

> "The natural healing force within each of us is the greatest force in getting well."
> —Hippocrates

Life moves fast, and so do injuries! Injuries do not typically happen while performing slow and controlled movements; they occur during fast movements, usually when you lose core control in an unpredicted event. In order to prepare your core for such incidents, you must challenge your contraction speed, muscle timing, and neuromuscular control. Initially, you should focus on strength and control with slow, fluid movements, as you need to develop the brakes before you can step on the gas. Once you develop control at slower speeds, then you can progress to a level comparable to normal, unpredictable daily life and sports.

In everyday activities, lifting with your spine in its natural, neutral position may not always be possible. For example, you may be in an awkward location or moving an oddly-shaped object. However, you can always make sure to pre-activate your core to provide support for your spine. This will eventually become automatic, and you will learn to gauge your core tone to match your task, whether you are lifting, throwing, or sprinting. A light task may only require gentle toning, whereas lifting heavier objects may require maximum bracing to support your spine.

Your speed of movement and your ability to generate forces, as well as your ability to react quickly to forces applied on your body from various directions, are key elements that can be achieved through medicine ball training. When your core muscles fire prior to your extremity muscles, this sequence of activation trains the core muscles to serve as prime movers and movement initiators, transferring force and motion to the extremity muscles to fine-tune the precision of your movement. By training your core to fire in these patterns consciously, the sequence of activation will eventually become automatic.

Exercising with medicine balls is an effective way of training your core muscles to work together to generate maximum torque, or rotational force, which develops the explosive power you need for vigorous activities such as jumping, running, throwing, hammering, and kicking. Medicine ball training allows complex movements to be performed with high torque acting on the core, which is necessary to perform swinging and twisting activities such as baseball, hockey, lacrosse, tennis, golf, and other rotational sports. In these activities, it is vital for the core to generate significant stabilizing forces during high angular velocity of your body parts. The ability of your core muscles to generate stabilizing force is necessary for optimal performance and injury prevention.

Medicine balls, also known as "exercise balls," "med balls," or "fitness balls," are weighted balls of various diameters and weights that make excellent tools for challenging your core stabilization muscles. Over three thousand years ago, Hippocrates stuffed animal skins and gave them to his patients to toss for "medicinal" purposes. In the seventeenth century, Persians were also known to have used similar balls for exercising their trunks. The term "medicine ball" dates back to the late 1800s, and these tools are still among the best for developing core stability by challenging neuromuscular control of the trunk and combining dynamic stabilization and mobilization of all segments of the kinetic chain in multiple planes.

Medicine balls range in size and weight, but you should start with a lightweight ball and slowly graduate to heavier ones to avoid compensations. A compensation is your body's attempt to make up for lack of control in one area by altering movement. More specifically, a compensation pattern is an alternate neuromuscular strategy your body unconsciously employs so you can complete a desired movement or task when the ideal natural neuromuscular strategy is no longer a viable option. This involves firing your muscles in different sequences, or utilizing structural reliance on your bones, ligaments, tendons, and joints. Patterns of compensation increase the risk of injury and damage to the body.

Safe lifting mechanics involve keeping heavy objects close to your body while maintaining your natural spinal alignment to minimize the forces that may injure your back. If you try to lift a heavy object away from your body, this increases the lever arm (the distance of the weight from your core), which increases the torque (the force amount multiplied by the lever arm) acting on your body. Medicine ball exercises take advantage of simple physics, training your core to ramp up the torque production in your core muscles by controlling a weighted ball at a distance from your center while twisting, turning, and bending in a wide array of angles.

To avoid compensations, the ball should be heavy enough to challenge you, but not so heavy to compromise your form. Be sure to hold the ball firmly and maintain control throughout the entire movement. If possible, use a mirror to provide visual feedback so you can optimize the fluidity of your motions. A good indicator of optimal form is the ability to pause with control at any point within the movement. Move with awareness and intention, rather than with momentum, which will funnel injurious forces throughout your body. When you can perform three sets of 12 repetitions with good form and ease, it is time to bump up the weight. Each medicine ball exercise must be refined with time and practice to integrate core control of the entire body for strength, agility, endurance, and balance for all activities of daily living and sports.

Core Med Ball Exercise #1: Med Ball Squat

Begin by standing tall in an upright position, holding the medicine ball in front of you with both arms extended, and with your feet slightly wider than hip-width apart. Squat by bending at your knees and hips until your knees are at an approximately 90-degree angle. Hinge at your hips, keep your back in its natural alignment, and keep your chest facing forward. Be sure to not let your knees cover your toes. Pause in this athletic position, with your weight resting slightly more on your heels, then drive through your heels to lift back to the starting position while raising the ball straight overhead to the sky.

Core Med Ball Exercise #2: Med Ball Anterior Posterior Lunges

Stand with a long, tall spine, holding a medicine ball with both arms straight overhead toward the sky. Bring the ball down toward your chest as you take a large step forward and lower down into a lunge position, allowing both knees to bend as your trunk sinks toward the floor. Don't allow your knees to collapse, or let your front knee move forward past your toes. Keep your trunk steady and controlled as you push yourself back to the starting position and raise the ball overhead. Repeat on the other side. For variation, try performing this exercise in reverse by stepping backward.

Core Med Ball Exercise #3: Med Ball Lateral Lunges

Stand tall with your feet hip-width apart, holding the medicine ball with both arms overhead. Take a wide step out to the side, flexing your hip and knee into a side lunge and driving your weight from the other extended leg. Make sure to keep your head and chest up. Then, extend through your bent leg to return to the starting position with controlled motion. Repeat on the other side.

Core Med Ball Exercise #4: Med Ball Diagonal Lunges

Stand tall with your feet hip-width apart, holding the medicine ball with both arms overhead. Take a wide step out diagonally to the side (at a 45-degree angle), flexing your hip and knee into a lunge and driving your weight from the other extended leg. Make sure to keep your head and chest up. Then, extend through your bent leg to return to the starting position with controlled motion. Repeat on the other side.

Core Med Ball Exercise #5: Med Ball Hip Drive

Stand tall with your feet hip-width apart, holding the medicine ball with both arms straight out in front of you. Avoid locking your elbows. Keep your chest facing forward and your head up as you balance on one leg and drive the other leg toward the ball. Be sure to ramp up your core activation before pushing the ball up in the air with your thigh. Catch the ball and repeat on the other leg.

Core Med Ball Exercise #6: Med Ball Trunk Twist

Stand tall while holding a medicine ball with both arms straight out in from of you, making sure not to lock your arms. Take a long step forward and lower down into a lunge position, allowing both knees to bend. Rotate your trunk toward your front leg as you move toward the floor. Do not allow your knees to collapse in, or let your front knee move forward past your toes. Keep your trunk steady and controlled as you push yourself back to the start position. Repeat on the other side.

Core Med Ball Exercise #7: Med Ball Core Revolutions

Stand tall with your legs hip-width apart, holding a medicine ball at chest-level with your arms bent at the elbows. In a fluid motion and with control of your trunk, pass the ball around your waist from one arm to the other and back around to the front. Try this clockwise and counterclockwise, then progress to variable motions such as circles or figure eights overhead.

Core Med Ball Exercises:

Table 4 illustrates seven core-empowering medicine ball exercises to further challenge your postural control and enhance your mind-core connectivity. Begin by simply performing the motions without any added weight. Move through these phases with focus on core control to establish stability, and progress with weight, speed, and repetitions, working up to three sets of 7-12 repetitions

Table 4. The Core Med Ball 7

Core Empowering Medicine Ball Exercises	Phase 1	Phase 2	Phase 3
Med Ball Squats			
Med Ball Anterior Posterior Lunges			
Med Ball Medial Lateral Lunges			
Med Ball Diagonal Lunges			
Med Ball Hip Drive			
Med Ball Trunk Twist			
Med Ball Core Revolutions			

Instability

> "My balance comes from instability."
> —Saul Bellow

The "pezzi ball," a large, puncture-resistant, air-filled gymnastics ball, was first developed in 1963 by Aquilino Cosani for playful exercise. Pezzi balls were first used in treatment programs for newborns and infants by Mary Quinton, a British physical therapist working in Switzerland. Dr. Susanne Klein-Vogelbach, the director at the Physical Therapy School in Basel, Switzerland, integrated the use of these therapeutic balls in physical therapy to treat children with neurological challenges. The term "Swiss ball" was used when American physical therapists began to use these techniques in North America after witnessing their benefits as instability devices in Switzerland.

This therapeutic ball is also known by a number of other names, including "balance ball," "birth ball," "body ball," "fitness ball," "gym ball," "gymnastic ball," "physio ball," "Pilates ball," "stability ball," "Swedish ball," "therapy ball," or "yoga ball." A modern adaptation of these therapeutic balls, BOSU™, has evolved as one of the most successful instability training devices that you can find at most gyms or physical therapy clinics. The term BOSU™ is derived from the phrase "both sides utilized," which represents the versatile use of this hemi-ball (half-ball) as a functional core stability trainer with a rounded side and a flat side. Wobble boards and natural surfaces (such as sand and gravel) also provide excellent alternatives as unstable training surfaces.

Stable balancing during everyday activities and athletic maneuvers demands pre-activation of the trunk to control all the parts of your body. The primary benefit of exercising on an unstable surface, as opposed to a hard, flat surface, is that the body responds by engaging more core musculature to maintain your balance. This means that you can train your body to recruit more of your core stabilizing muscles that wouldn't be activated by training on regular, flat surfaces.

Instability exercises facilitate the production of neuromuscular engrams, or memory pathways, that train your core to rapidly react to external forces of unwanted motions or unanticipated perturbations, like when you are pushed, or step in a hole. These memory pathways are like software programs in your nervous system that pre-activate and synchronize your core musculature to rapidly react to motion and perturbation, which occur too fast for you to actually think about correcting your body position. Developing these memory pathways will keep you centered, and more aware of and responsive to your body's position, improving performance and preventing loss of stability to spare you from injury. So, get on the ball and amp up your core response!

Core-Stabilizing Exercise #1: Stability Bug

The Stability Bug is performed on your back, as you lie on top of an unstable object (like a Pezzi ball). Find your balance in an outstretched position with one arm reaching overhead. Take turns alternately raising your arms up toward the sky, synchronizing your movements with opposite leg motion and lifting to a position of 90 degrees at your hip and knee. Try an advanced version of the stability bug by keeping both legs straight throughout the alternate synchronous motion. To further challenge your core, flail your limbs at varying speeds and in various directions to mimic the unpredictable motions of life.

Core-Stabilizing Exercise #2: Stability Bridge

Begin the Stability Bridge by lying on your back with your knees comfortably bent and feet on an unstable object. Press your feet into the object as you lift your trunk up from the lowest vertebra to the highest, forming a long, straight line from your shoulders to your knees.

Lengthen through the front of your hips, then slowly lower down one vertebra at a time from the neck to the tailbone. Increase the intensity by squeezing a ball or block between your knees, or by adding resistance bands around your thighs. Experiment with moving the unstable surface from your feet to under your upper back. Additional variations include lifting each leg alternately off the object, and/or standing up on your toes.

Core-Stabilizing Exercise #3: Stability Bird Dog

The Stability Bird Dog exercise is performed in the quadruped position (on your hands and knees), first with your forearms on an unstable surface. Raise an arm and the opposite leg straight out to form one line with your trunk, making sure not to sway or twist your pelvis. Maintain control of your trunk as you switch arms and legs. Add variable arm and leg motions to further ramp up the core muscle activation, or even resistance with bands. You may also shift your weight forward through your arm on the unstable surface, floating the weightbearing knee off the ground to provide additional destabilizing forces, which increases your core muscle recruitment. To further challenge your core, try placing the unstable surface under your knees.

Core-Stabilizing Exercise #4: Stability Plank

Position your body face-down with your forearms on the ground and feet on an unstable surface. With your elbows directly under your shoulders and your fingers pointing forward, prop your body up off the ground. Your head should stay in a neutral alignment, with your gaze toward the floor to avoid neck strain. Focus on keeping your trunk rigid in a neutral spine position, or a straight line from head to toe, with no sagging or arching. To advance the plank, progress to weight-bearing through the hands instead of forearms (you should be in push-up position), and by incorporating shoulder taps to the opposite shoulder to increase core activity and stabilize while balancing on one arm. For further core challenge, lift one leg at a time to promote increased activation of the core musculature.

Core-Stabilizing Exercise #5: Stability Side Plank

Begin the stability side plank on your side, with your legs fully extended and stacked on top of each other, and your feet resting on an unstable surface. Use your elbow and your forearm to prop your body up in a straight line from your head to your toes. Keep your core tight and your neck in line with your body. Avoid raising or dropping your head. Be aware of your hip position, as sagging or dropping indicates fatigue, at which point the exercise should be stopped. Repeat on the other side. For a dynamic progression, try lifting your upper leg (and even your arm) toward the sky, then back to the starting position while maintaining trunk alignment. Advance to weightbearing through your hand instead of your forearm.

Core-Stabilizing Exercise #6: Superhero

The Superhero is performed lying down with your belly on top of an unstable surface with your arms and legs outstretched. Keep your limbs straight, but not locked. Engage your core as you lift one arm and the opposite leg a few inches toward the sky, keeping them straight. Repeat with the other arm and leg. Lengthen through your spine, and make sure not to shrug your shoulders. Advance the Superhero by lifting all your limbs toward the sky as high as you can, again keeping them straight but not locked.

Core-Stabilizing Exercise #7: Stability Squat

Step carefully onto an unstable surface, with the support of a countertop or sturdy chair within reach. Stand as tall as possible with your feet hip-width apart, and your arms in front of you to maintain your balance. Keeping your back in its natural alignment, tilt your trunk forward as you hinge at your hips to sit back into an imaginary chair until your thighs are parallel to the floor. Make sure to keep your knees behind your toes. Pause in this athletic position, with your weight resting slightly more on the heels to engage your core, while your trunk is elongated forward and up. Drive through the heels to lift back to the starting position. To further challenge your core, progress to a single leg squat, as you extend your non-weightbearing leg in front of you.

Core Stabilizing Exercises:

Table 5 illustrates seven core stabilizing exercises that may be performed on any unstable surface, including foam, cork, wobble boards, BOSU™, or pezzi balls. Have fun and get creative by experimenting with your own unstable surface, whether it's a kayak, a sailboat, an air mattress, or your kid's bounce house. Begin with phase 1 and progress to phase 2 for optimal core muscle recruitment and stabilization, working up to three sets of 7-12 repetitions with at least a five second hold for each, and holding the last repetition for thirty seconds.

Table 5. The Core Stabilizing 7

Core Stabilizers	Phase 1	Phase 2
Stability Bug		
Stability Bridge		
Stability Bird Dog		
Stability Plank		
Stability Side Plank		
Superhero		
Stability Squat		

Plyometrics

"Jump, and you will find out how to unfold your wings as you fall."
—Ray Bradbury

Power is a product of force and velocity. This basic principle of physics is important for core empowerment. Once force (or core strength) is established, velocity (or speed) may be incorporated with quick movements to further challenge and empower your core. Daily activities and sports require movements that combine both strength and speed to create power. Plyometrics, or jump training exercises, assist in the development of core stability and your ability to generate power in everything you do. Plyometric principles have been used for many decades in the training of Ukrainian and Russian athletes.

Yuri Verkhoshansky, a Russian track and field coach, originated the concept of "jump training," or "shock training." He was the first to recognize the amortization (transition) phase, which is the very brief moment in a jump when you transition from descending down into the jump to ascending upwards with explosive power. This is called the "stretch-shorten cycle," when a muscle actively stretches, then is immediately shortened. The faster this transition occurs, the higher you can jump. In the 1960s, Verkhoshsansky began publishing his methodical jump research, in which he had athletes drop from a box, land briefly as they absorbed the shock, and then immediately jump as high as possible, higher than ever before.

This exciting phenomenon was incorporated into the training of athletes all over the world for enhanced performance. In 1975, former Olympic athlete and Purdue University track coach Fred Wilt studied and applied Verkoshansky's work with his athletes and described this form of training as "plyometrics." The word "plyometrics" is actually a derivation of the Latin words "pilo," meaning "to increase," and "metric," which means "to measure." Consequently, the goal of plyometrics is "to increase measurement."

In sports performance outcomes, measurements can include height, distance, or speed. A faster amortization phase results in more efficient use of the stretch-shorten cycle in muscles, and more effective absorption of the forces, which then translates to greater power. The goals of plyometric training are to decrease this transition phase, and to allow safe adaptation to the rigors of explosive daily activities and sports while maintaining focus on proper techniques and biomechanics.

We have now recognized the importance of jumping, not just for performance, but as a critical component of injury prevention programs. Plyometric training induces beneficial neuromuscular adaptations in the core musculature, your kinetic chain, and your nervous system to enhance dynamic stability. Muscle pre-activation significantly increases after plyometric training to enhance dynamic restraint throughout your body and functional core stability.

Plyometric exercises are advanced core exercises that should be attempted only after core awareness and strength have been established, and are geared toward highly trained athletes, or people in peak physical condition without musculoskeletal problems. However, these same exercises may be modified with reduced stress on your muscles, tendons, and joints by performing them on a trampoline or in water, beginning in deeper water and progressing to shallower levels. Try plyometrics in the ocean, a lake, a pond, or even a river with a sandy bottom, and hop your way to an explosively powerful core.

Core Plyometric Exercise #1: Sky Hops

Start with your feet hip-width apart, toes pointing forward and arms reaching straight up. Lengthen by stretching through the crown of your head toward the sky. Gently squat down until your knees slightly bend, then press up through your heels to jump up and down as quickly as possible, landing softly without letting your knees fall in toward each other.

Core Plyometric Exercise #2: Scissor Hops

Stand in a split stance with one leg forward and the other leg back. Your feet should be approximately one to two feet apart, with weight distributed equally on both legs. Jump straight up into the air as high as possible, reversing your legs in the air and landing with your feet in the opposite positions. Keep your knees soft to avoid locking them.

Core Plyometric Exercise #3: Lunge Hops

Stand in a split stance with one leg forward and the other leg back. Your feet should be approximately two to three feet apart, with weight distributed equally on both legs. Bend your knees and lower your body, bringing your back knee as close to the ground as you can while maintaining good control. Jump straight up as high as you can, reversing your legs in the air and landing with your feet in the opposite positions. Make sure to land with your front knee behind your toes.

Core Plyometric Exercise #4: Anterior Posterior Hops

Start by standing behind an object that you can clear on a jump. If you are unaccustomed to jumping, try using a piece of tape to mark the ground instead. Stand as tall as possible with your feet hip-width apart, and your arms in front of you to maintain your balance. Dip into a squat position while keeping your back in its natural alignment as you quickly sit back into an imaginary chair as low as you can and explode quickly upward and forward, landing gently on both feet. Immediately squat down, then push upward and back to the starting position. Make sure to keep your knees behind your toes.

Core Plyometric Exercise #5: Medial Lateral Hops

Start by standing to the side of an object that you can clear on a jump. (Again, if you are unaccustomed to jumping, try using a piece of tape to mark the ground instead.) Stand as tall as possible with your feet hip-width apart, and your arms in front of you to maintain your balance. Dip into a squat position while keeping your back in its natural alignment as you sit back into an imaginary chair as low as you can, then quickly explode upward and sideways before landing gently on both feet. Immediately squat down and push upward and back to the starting position. Make sure to keep your knees behind your toes.

Core Plyometric Exercise #6: Horizon to Sky Hops

Stand as tall as possible with your feet hip-width apart and your arms stretched out in front of you to maintain balance. Dip into a squat position while keeping your back in its natural alignment as you sit back into an imaginary chair as low as you can, then quickly explode upward and forward before landing gently on both feet. Immediately squat down and push upward as you reach for the sky, jumping as high as you can. Make sure to keep your knees behind your toes. Return to the starting position. If you have the space, perform the reps without delay, moving forward as far and as high as you can when you jump.

Core Plyometric Exercise #7: Inchworm Hops

Position your body face-down in a push-up position, with your elbows directly under your shoulders. Your head should stay in a neutral alignment, with your gaze toward the floor, to avoid neck strain. Focus on keeping your trunk rigid in a neutral spine position, or a straight line from head to toe, with no sagging or arching. Transfer all of your weight to your hands, bend your knees as you hop your feet forward, then kick your feet back out before repeating without delay.

Core Plyometric Exercises:

Table 6 illustrates seven core plyometric exercises. For all plyometrics, try to roll on the balls of your feet to minimize ground reaction forces. You can start by performing these exercises with supportive athletic shoes that have good shock absorption before trying them barefoot. Recent evidence shows that plyometrics performed barefoot in water or sand provide less strain on muscles, bones, and connective tissue, but offer the same benefits of traditional plyometrics on a firm surface. Begin with small hops and progress by increasing height and repetitions. Focus on speed, power, and soft landings.

Table 6. The Core Plyometric 7

Core Plyometrics	Phase 1	Phase 2
Sky Hops		
Scissor Hops		
Lunge Hops		
Anterior Posterior Hops		
Medial Lateral Hops		
Horizon to Sky Hops		
Inchworm Hops		

Suspension

"You are much stronger than
you think you are!"
—Spiderman

A spider hanging from its thread may remain completely motionless, instead of rotating or swinging back and forth. We can learn a thing or two from these amazing arachnids. If you have ever watched these fascinating little creatures hanging out, you would notice that they can suspend, motionless, on a vertical thread with complete stability, and they can always recover balance after any type of disturbance (such as a gust of wind or pouring rain). Maybe that's why these stupefying, suspended stabilizers are all core with skinny legs?

In all seriousness, suspension training, or hanging like a spider, is an amazing way to beef up your own core muscle activation and control. Suspension exercise is a form of core stability training that uses ropes or straps with a single point anchor, and your own body weight for resistance. This core-training strategy was first developed by ancient South Americans, before becoming popular among the Navy Seals. Recently, it was commercialized with the TrX™ (Total Resistance Exercise) you can find at almost every gym.

Using functional movements and dynamic positioning, suspension core exercises incorporate some basic principles of physics, including Newton's law of gravitation force vectors and Galileo's pendulum principle. A pendulum is a weight suspended from a pivot point, like a spider on a thread, so that it can swing freely. When the weight is displaced from its resting, equilibrium position, the force of gravity will accelerate the weight back to the equilibrium position, causing it to oscillate back and forth.

During suspension exercises, your core is trained to reflexively sense, react to, and control the oscillatory forces. These principles of physics are further applied by changing the angle of the straps or ropes, and thereby the forces on the body. The combination of these forces creates gravitational potential energy (energy stored based on your body's position) and kinetic energy (energy of your body's motion) while your center of gravity is suspended. Think of an arrow that is pulled back in a bow with potential energy, which is converted to kinetic energy when it is released. The pendulum of the single point anchor system converts this energy to resistance, which challenges and trains the stability of your core and your entire body's chain.

Although suspension exercises are used to develop strength and stability to generate more core power for high-level athletes, these exercises may be easily modified for beginners, seniors, or people recovering from injuries. Beginners can perform these safely by moving their body positions closer in relation to the anchor point, limiting the excursion of the exercise, or by adjusting the base of support to a wider stance. To advance the difficulty of suspension exercises, increase the stability demands on your core by training at a greater angle of pull, or even advancing to single-limb balancing.

Scientific studies have shown that during suspension workouts, activity levels of the core muscles are higher compared to exercises performed on stable or unstable support surfaces. So, have fun "hanging out" and developing your super-spidey core power!

Core Suspension Exercise #1: Side Crunch

Begin by standing in an upright position, facing to one side and holding the handles of your resistance bands with both hands overhead and your elbows bent. Stand with good posture, aligning your ears, shoulders, hips, knees, and ankles in one vertical line. Keep your knees soft so that your muscles are active, but your knees are not locked. Slowly sink your hips out to your side until you feel a stretch along the side of your body and hold for five seconds. Repeat on the other side.

Core Suspension Exercise #2: Roll Out

Begin in a kneeling position, holding a handle in each hand with an overhand grip at chest height. Keeping your arms straight but not locked, lean forward as far as you are able for five seconds. Reverse the movement to return to the starting position and repeat. Make sure to keep your movements slow and controlled during the exercise. Do not arch your back or shrug your shoulders.

Core Suspension Exercise #3: Suspended Planks

Begin in a tall kneeling position in front of the straps. Place one foot in each of the straps, then place your hands directly below your shoulders and raise up into a plank. Drop onto one elbow at a time. Hold for five seconds, then raise up onto your hands, one at a time. Try to minimize rotation during the exercise, and do not allow your back to arch.

Core Suspension Exercise #4: Suspended Side Planks

Begin on one side with your hips in line with the anchor and place your feet in the straps. Use your hand (or elbow, to modify) to push yourself up. Lift your hips by pressing into the foot cradles. Look straight ahead and hold the plank for five seconds; rest, reset, and lift back up. Rest and repeat while lying on the other side. Try to keep hips and shoulders vertically stacked, and your bottom shoulder away from your ear.

Core Suspension Exercise #5: Suspended Crunch

Begin in a tall kneeling position in front of the straps. Place one foot in each of the straps, then place your hands directly below your shoulders to raise up into a plank. Maintaining your plank position, bring both knees toward your chest. Hold for five seconds, then return to the plank position and repeat. Make sure to keep your abdominals engaged and your trunk parallel to the ground. Do not let your back arch or rotate during the exercise.

Core Suspension Exercise #6: Climber

Begin by kneeling on both knees in front of the straps. Place one foot in each of the straps, then place your hands directly below your shoulders and raise up into a plank. Maintaining your plank position, bring one knee toward your chest. Hold for five seconds, then return to the plank position and repeat with your opposite leg. Make sure to keep your abdominals engaged and your trunk parallel to the ground. Do not let your back arch or rotate during the exercise.

Core Suspension Exercise #7: Pike

Begin again by kneeling on both knees in front of the straps. Place one foot in each of the straps, then place your hands directly below your shoulders and raise up into a plank. Maintaining a natural, neutral spine, hike your hips up for five seconds, then return to the plank position. When you hike your hips, your body forms an upside-down "V" with your spine in its neutral alignment, and your knees straight but soft. Keep your abdominals engaged and your trunk parallel to the ground. Do not let your back arch or rotate during the exercise.

Core Suspension Exercises:

Table 7 illustrates seven core suspension exercises that may be performed with ropes or TrX™ (Total Resistance Exercise) straps. Progress through these phases slowly, focusing on core control to establish stability throughout your kinetic chain. Begin with small movements and work up to three sets of 7-12 repetitions each, with sustained positioning for five seconds each, and holding the last repetition for thirty seconds.

Table 7. The Core Suspension 7

Core Suspension	Phase 1	Phase 2
Side Crunch		
Roll Out		
Suspended Planks		
Suspended Side Plank		
Suspended Crunch		
Climber		
Pike		

Seeds for Thought

- On a scale of 1–10 (with 10 being the best), how would you rate your current balancing abilities?
- How do you think improving your balance could benefit your performance and ability to perform daily tasks safely?
- Which exercises did you find most challenging?
- How did it feel to perform squats, lunges, and other exercises with a medicine ball compared to performing those exercises without the extra weight?
- What types of real-world activities will practicing these functional exercises improve?

CHAPTER 12

Empowerment: The Core-Flourishing Phase

"We never know how high we are
Till we are called to rise;
And then, if we are true to plan,
Our statures touch the skies."
—Emily Dickinson

We've now arrived at the part of the Core BASE Guide where you get to choose your own core-empowering activities. Creating and maintaining a healthy core requires a commitment to living a healthy lifestyle and engaging regularly in fun activities that challenge your core and nurture your spirit. You deserve to have plenty of fun, excitement, and play in your life, and we know that incorporating these kinds of activities will dramatically improve your mental, emotional, and physical health. In this chapter, I'll introduce you to several alternative philosophies and activities that have been proven by science to be highly beneficial to your health and core.

Your job in the Empowerment phase is to choose the activities that nurture your soul and spirit, and bring you joy while improving your core stability and fitness. This will allow you to continuously improve your core awareness, control, and health throughout your lifetime, instead of staying stuck in a cycle of moving from one workout plan to another without seeing the results you want. True empowerment comes from exploration, so explore your own path to empowerment with exciting adventures and challenges.

If you've ever watched cat and mouse cartoons like Tom and Jerry, Jinx, or Ren and Stimpy, you no doubt admired the brave little mice who dare to go out and explore while their predator is out of sight, channeling their fear into challenge and pushing their limits into the danger zone. Humans are programmed the same way as all living creatures, with an intrinsic drive to explore, empower ourselves, and learn strategies to protect ourselves. Yet sometimes, this drive gets overridden by the stressors of daily life and we forget to embrace our innate mindset of playfulness, imagination, adventure, and challenge. Empower your core by exploring your relationship with the universe around you and engaging in activities that improve your fitness while making you happy. Fitness should not be boring!

As Eleanor Roosevelt said, "You must do the things you think you cannot do." Dare yourself to try a new activity, such as paddle boarding, surfing, mountain biking, snowboarding, trail running, or rock climbing. Do not fear the storm, for you will learn to sail your ship through wind and wave. This is not only beneficial for your physical core, but also your mind. You will become centered and whole by developing new pathways that connect your brain to your core in a happy flow, where you are completely engaged, absorbed, and empowered in mind, body, and spirit.

Many of my patients have asked me what kinds of fun activities they can practice to work their cores while building strength, other than just hitting the gym. I usually direct them toward core-empowering activities such as Pilates, yoga, martial arts, dance, and other fun sports in the wonders of nature, like surfing or skiing. The benefits of trying such alternative and complementary practices for core empowerment are now being recognized by the scientific community, and we'll explore those benefits in more detail below. You will reap the rewards of trying new things by experiencing more fun, joy, and a healthier core, so don't be afraid to try something new just because you don't know how, or you think it might be too difficult or awkward to learn. You'll never know until you try it!

Pilates

"The mind, when housed within a healthful body, possesses a glorious sense of power."
—Joseph Pilates

Millions of people around the world have used Joseph Pilates' specialized exercise to develop their core "powerhouse," with 11 million practitioners and 14,000 instructors in the United States alone.

German-born Pilates first developed his technique back in the mid-1900s. He grew up a fragile boy, weakened by rheumatic fever, rickets, and asthma, which spurred his passion for exercise, health, and wellness, and his life studies in Eastern mind-body arts, anatomy, bodybuilding, boxing, wrestling, gymnastics, and martial arts.

At the outbreak of World War I, Pilates was interned as an enemy alien in England, and although not formally educated, he began acting as a physiotherapist to his fellow injured internees. Pilates invented his own strengthening equipment by rigging patients' bedsprings to bedposts, headboards, and footboards. These homemade designs were early models of the universal reformer and trapeze table, the benchmark apparatuses of today's Pilates studios.

Joseph Pilates philosophized that holistic health, a balanced lifestyle, and core exercise activate brain cells to stimulate the mind and impact the body. Recently, science has substantiated that exercise improves cognition and executive function of the brain, supporting Pilates' theories and approach to health and injury prevention.

Studies now show that many Pilates techniques align, lengthen, and protect the spine, and can effectively develop core muscle strength. By combining mental focus with mindful breathing and precise, rhythmical movements, you too can develop greater core and trunk muscle strength that provides alignment and protection of the spine for skilled movements with better balance and coordination. These techniques are loved by dancers, athletes, and all who are looking to strengthen and tone their bodies. Pilates' techniques are also beneficial for those suffering from back pain or recovering from injuries, and have been shown to help reduce stress and musculoskeletal pain, improve flexibility, and promote better posture and relaxation.

The traditional, classical approach of "Contrology" (as Pilates referred to his own exercise method) adheres to his original work, which teaches abdominal exercises in a "posterior tilt." This is when you completely press your lower spine into the ground while lying on your back, creating a tuck in your pelvis. Contemporary Pilates is based on his original ideas, but has been modernized by adjusting the exercises based on new biomechanical research.

Contemporary Pilates teaches exercises in a "neutral pelvis" position, or the position your spine is in when standing upright in a healthy, natural posture. While exercising the core in the neutral spine and lying on your back, as you have learned in the Core BASE Guide, the lower spine will have space between the ground and the back, and your hips and pubic bone will be level in one plane. Modern Pilates, based on the century-old principles of Contrology, has evolved to integrate the current evidence-based principles with traditional core training techniques.

Yoga

"Yoga is the journey of the self, through the self, to the self."
—The Gita

More than 15 percent of adults (36.7 million people) in the United States have begun their journey to core empowerment with yoga, which represents an increase of over 16 million since 2012. In fact, three out of every four yogis and yoginis are relatively new to the practice, having started within the last five years. The rapid rise of yoga practice is spanning across all age groups and ethnicities. Yogic philosophy and practice combine breathing exercises, physical postures, and meditation to calm the nervous system, activate the core, and balance the body, mind, and spirit.

Five thousand years of ancient Hindu texts and traditions identify the core, or "solar plexus," as the place where our personal identities, confidence, and power are stored. The scientific community is recognizing the importance of this alternative philosophy, with approximately 55 percent of physical therapists regularly using yoga as a common form of alternative strength training, and to address various musculoskeletal problems.

Yoga exercises can be varied and scaled to fit your age, fitness level, and medical profile. Recent scientific research supports the effectiveness of yoga for alleviating chronic pain, as well as the premise that yoga brings balance and health to the physical, mental, emotional, and spiritual core with an eightfold path for a disciplined, purposeful, healthy life.

The word "yoga" is derived from the Sanskrit root "yuj", which means to unite. The ultimate goal of yoga is to unite your mind-body-spirit to achieve self-empowerment with strength, stability, and resilience. Yoga is also a separation or disentanglement from anything hindering your path to empowerment, so you can attain "moksha," meaning liberation or freedom, and cultivate a calm, inner balance regardless of external circumstances.

Yoga practice exemplifies the ancient Eastern philosophy of Yin and Yang, a concept of dualism in which seemingly opposite forces are actually complimentary and interdependent within our bodies and the natural world. Yin qualities are internal, passive, and downward, whereas Yang qualities are external, dynamic, and upward. The Yang aspect of yoga promotes strength and cardiovascular fitness, whereas the Yin aspect of yoga promotes flexibility and mindfulness to ground you and calm your nervous system. Today's fast-paced world promotes a Yang-oriented lifestyle of excitement and productivity, yet may lead to burnout and health issues if not balanced with Yin, or the quiet and calm within your mind-body-spirit.

Yoga postures comprise simple body movements with bends, twists, and inversions while standing, sitting, kneeling, lying down, or resting on hands and knees. The practice of "asanas" aligns, strengthens, and balances the body, while enhancing dynamic control of core-stabilizing muscles. Pranayama is the yogic practice of breath training. The word "prana," meaning "energy" or "life source," is the very essence that keeps us alive, as well as the energy in the universe around us. Pranayama, or "breath control," is used to nourish and energize the body, calm the mind, and engage the core. Although ancient yogis did not have the scientific studies to support their practice, they recognized the important connection between breath, emotions, and health.

With experience, yoga strategies may be incorporated into everyday life so you can focus on the present moment, where sensations and sounds don't easily distract the mind. Dharana, meaning "focused concentration," draws awareness of your breathing and core using the strategies of Focused Attention Meditation. Dhyana, or "meditative absorption," utilizes an approach similar to Open Monitoring Meditation to achieve objective, non-judgmental, and non-reactive observation of breath, posture, and core function in the present moment. And finally, Samadhi, meaning "see equally" or "realization," is a state of ecstasy similar to what you experience in Transcendental Meditation. Achieving this feeling of bliss and fulfillment is the highest state of consciousness and union with your highest reality and the universe, which is the ultimate goal of yoga practice for core empowerment.

Martial Arts

"Understand that the essence of martial arts is not the art itself, but
what's hidden deep within yourself."
—Gogen Yamaguchi

"Kim, are you ok?!" I gasped, and as I reached out to help my
friend off the mat, a lock of her golden curls fell from my trembling
hand. For a moment, I forgot the gymnasium full of eyes beaming on
us, and the cheers of our classmates fell silent. Aside from wrestling
my brothers as a child, this final examination of our physical education
elective, Jujitsu (also spelled Jiu Jitsu), was the first time I ever fought
another person, much less flipped one over onto the ground. As Kim
smiled and popped back up, I immediately felt relief, and my initial
apprehension transformed into a sense of empowerment. I had utilized
the principles of harnessing core energy that our instructor helped us
develop over the semester to actually toss my buddy over my shoulder
like a sack of potatoes!

Years later, I was again introduced to these principles through the
International Silat Foundation at Yale University. Silat is an indigenous
martial art from maritime Southeast Asia, surmised to have been
originated by a woman who witnessed a fight between a tiger and a
hawk. By mimicking the animals' movements, she was able to fend
off a group of men that had attacked her. Silat shares similar core
principles with other martial arts, including Jujitsu, Tai Chi, Karate,
and Tae Kwon Do.

"Ju" can be translated to "pliable" or "yielding." "Jutsu" can be
translated to mean "art" or "technique," and is based on the principle of
manipulating an attacker's force against them, rather than confronting
it with your own force. Jujitsu, developed in fifteenth century Japan,
promotes core awareness as the great equalizer of size and strength,
using leverage and physics to level this disparity. As I did, you too can
learn to flip and roll opponents twice your size, giving you confidence
to accomplish things you never would have imagined.

Of all the martial arts that empower the core, Tai Chi is the
most scientifically studied and has been shown to improve balance,
cognitive function, and postural control through slow, meditative body
movements, originally designed for self-defense and promoting inner
peace and calm. Tai Chi masters are also able to throw an attacker

effortlessly to the floor using core energy and control. This is reflected in the Tai Chi saying that "ounces can deflect thousands of pounds," as a defender can use a small amount of energy to neutralize the far greater external force of an attacker.

Karate evolved from East Asia over a period of centuries and became systematized in the seventeenth century as an art of self-defense through mind-core control. Modern Karate emphasizes the psychological elements of perseverance, fearlessness, virtue, and leadership skills. Taekwondo also has ancient roots that date all the way back to 50 B.C. in Korea. "Tae" means "to kick," "kwon" means "to punch with the hand," and "do" means "a method of doing something," thus Taekwondo utilizes the strategy of core control of upper and lower limb high velocity maneuvers for self-defense.

Taekwondo is characterized by its emphasis on fast, high jumps and spinning kick techniques, which challenge the core with single-leg balancing of postural control by incorporating dynamic extremity movements. To facilitate fast, turning kicks, Taekwondo adopts stances that are narrower and taller than the broader, wider stances used by Karate, which challenges your core to provide stability with agility. The emphasis on speed and agility is a defining characteristic of martial arts, as the kinetic energy of a strike increases exponentially with the speed of the strike, but increases only linearly with the mass of the striking object. In other words, speed is more important than size in terms of generating power.

The common skill of all experienced martial artists is their ability to harness and generate core energy as the powerhouse, or engine for all limb movement. To understand the phenomenon of core power generation, it is helpful to analyze the proportions of the human body, as great thinkers have done for centuries. Over two millenniums ago, "The Man in the Circle and Square," described and illustrated by Vitruvius (best known from Leonardo da Vinci's famous drawing), placed a human body directly in the center of a circle and a square.

Vitruvius recognized that "the navel is naturally the exact center of the body. For if a man lies on his back with hands and feet outspread, and the center of a circle is placed on his navel, his fingers and toes will be touched by the circumference. Also, a square will be found described within the figure, in the same way as a round figure is produced. For if we measure from the sole of the foot to the top of the head, and apply the measure to the outstretched hands, the breadth will be found equal to the height, just like sites which are squared by rule."

Da Vinci acknowledged these symmetrical, complementary proportions of the core in relation to the human body in his meticulous studies and famous drawing, "Vitruvian Man." He drew upper body and lower body triangles that met at the center of the body, and recognized this as the reservoir of energy production and transfer throughout the body. Our biomechanical studies now support the work of this Renaissance man.

In martial arts, the larger muscles of the lower body (Da Vinci's lower triangle) generate power, and the center transfers the power to the upper body (the upper triangle), while providing stability and rooting. Newton's third law of motion states that "every action has an equal and opposite reaction." Following this principle, when the lower limbs push against the ground, the ground pushes against the lower limbs. Proper rooting in the ground maximizes the potential of your body to transfer power from your limbs through your core. Without proper grounding, you would recoil from forces applied against you.

Successful grounding is dependent upon core bracing. With core bracing, all the muscles of your trunk contract to stabilize your trunk isometrically (without moving your spine), tightening your core circumferentially as if to protect you from a punch to the abdomen. Core bracing quickly generates maximum intraabdominal pressure, which decreases perturbation of the trunk to a sudden load. This principle is important in injury prevention, especially when your trunk is exposed to unexpected, heavy loads. Intraabdominal pressure is also important for core muscle force development. Without core bracing, the transfer of power from and through the core is diminished. Poor core muscle firing patterns send a red flag to your nervous system to decrease the force produced through an unstable core. Harnessing energy through a stable core to maximize power production is the key principle of martial arts, and the common element of these disciplines for core empowerment, injury prevention, and rehabilitation.

The phenomenon of core empowerment through martial arts may not only be explained by physics, but also by neurophysiology. We have discussed the detrimental effects of a chronically overactive sympathetic nervous system on your health, but it is important to note that the adrenal surge that comes with the activation of your sympathetic nervous system is beneficial when you want to optimally access power reserves for peak performance. This concept dates back to the Viking "berserkers," who would deliberately harness the energy of the sympathetic surge with a frenzy of head clashing, shield-biting, roaring, and howling to psych themselves up in a frenzy prior to battle. But you don't have to go berserk to use mind power for boosting energy, as is evident in athletic competition. When the stakes are high, we usually perform at our best. A common principle of all martial arts is learning how to access mind power through mental discipline in order to harness energy. Yet mind power alone cannot explain the stories we hear of superhuman feats in strength during emergency situations, like when a mother lifts a car off of her trapped baby. This is when we as scientists recognize that there is so much more to learn about the power of the spirit and metaphysical factors in summoning superhuman strength.

Dance

"Life isn't about waiting for the storm to pass. It's about learning to dance in the rain."
—Vivian Greene

Dance is the most fundamental of the arts, and a wonderful way to incorporate musical and bodily movements in your journey to core empowerment. Although dance has always been an important part of all cultures, it was not until the twenty-first century that this form of expression evolved as a complementary medicine recognized for health benefits, including improved flexibility, muscle strength and tone, endurance, balance, spatial awareness, coordination, cardiovascular conditioning, and general well-being.

Dance provides a rhythmic stimulation that enhances your mind-body connection. Complementary practices of martial arts provide a ritualized, structured form of dance, yet mindful movement in any and all forms of dance empowers the core and should be encouraged from infancy. As a young girl, Ukrainian dancing challenged my core with systematic progressions of stepping, spinning, multi-directional dynamic movements, and acrobatics. These types of challenges develop control of postural alignment with an everchanging base of support.

Dancers learn to maintain a vertical orientation of the trunk throughout these multi-directional movements, which develops important neuromuscular patterns in the body's software. These updates to the nervous system's software are integral for balance, as they challenge the brain to form new circuitry. This updated circuitry improves connectivity, speed, and reaction times to keep you centered and stable in a world full of motion. That's why it's not surprising that recent evidence shows improved core stability and fewer injuries in dancers.

Dancers are notorious for having perfect posture, but you don't have to be a professional to learn to be graceful, centered, and powerful. Research shows dance improves your posture, mood, and outlook on life. Choose tap, jazz, hip hop, ballroom, or freestyle to empower your core physically and emotionally with fun and groove.

Music

"Rhythm and harmony find their way into the inward places of the soul."
—Plato

Music echoes the rhythm of life in major and minor keys, crescendos and diminuendos, tensions and resolutions, dynamics and phrasing, pauses and silent interludes, and temporal sequences and climaxes that reveal the nature of your core with an accuracy that language cannot convey. The link between music and health is documented in the writing of ancient philosophers, yet only recently has it permeated neuroscientific research.

Over two thousand years ago, Plato recognized that music played in various modes could arouse different thoughts and emotions. Yet, the formal profession of music therapy was only established after the world wars, when musicians played for veterans to soothe both physical and emotional suffering and heal them with the joy of song. The patients' extraordinarily positive body and mind responses spurred a formal college curriculum in the 1940s, establishing music therapy as an organized clinical profession in the United States.

Scientists are now recognizing the ability of music and song to enhance brain development and neuroplasticity, specifically improving memory, language, I.Q., and visuospatial skills. Even just humming a tune has the power to soothe and calm you, and has recently been shown to improve circulation, oxygenation, and relaxation, lowering heart rate and blood pressure, as well as boosting oxytocin, the natural "love" hormone.

Musical rhythms also promote enhanced core muscle activation during singing due to rapid inhalation and expanding lung volume. Long exhalations increase the intra-abdominal and sub-glottal pressure-generating capacity of the diaphragm, abdominal muscles, and pelvic floor. These adaptations have been associated with improvements in sound power spectrum and have implications for voice quality, as commonly advocated by classical singing teachers and professionals. Choose the song you love and send it from your core, using your body as your instrument!

You might want to empower your body, mind, and spirit by learning a musical instrument. Whether you are pounding some rhythm and blues on the piano, blowing some sweet soul into a saxophone, or thrashing out some pent-up emotions on the drums, making music will strengthen your body and soul. Playing any instrument develops mindful breathing, postural alignment, and core awareness and control.

Musicians have great postural awareness. This might be the result of years of reminders from music instructors, or simply due to the fact that good posture naturally develops the most effective and efficient breathing and sound. Wind instruments especially encourage relaxed inhalation and controlled, precise, and sometimes forceful exhalations that can give your inner core a great workout! Taking in deep breaths teaches your diaphragm and inner core muscles to engage at full lung capacity at varying speeds and force. Instruments that require forceful exhalation, like a tuba or trumpet, further engage these muscles to properly support your sound while developing your mind and core.

Making music enhances coordination, forces you to focus on controlled motions of your muscles, and requires attentive, precise repetitions at varying speeds to build new neural pathways in your brain and body. Learning how to calm your nervous system so it can function well under pressure during performances is a useful skill that carries over to other stressful life situations. Similar to Focused Attention Meditation for establishing self-awareness, playing or singing your heart out will center you with good postural alignment, healthy breathing, and core awareness!

Laughter

"Laugh my friend, for laughter ignites a fire within the pit of your
belly, and awakens your being."
—Stella McCartney

Light up your face with a smile, chuckle with your whole belly, and
let laughter empower your core. "Duchenne" smiling (named for the
nineteenth century French doctor), or "smizing" with all the muscles
of your face—including your lips, cheeks, and eyes—has recently been
demonstrated by MRI to provide feedback that stimulates the brain.
This neurofeedback acts as a mood booster and stress buster. The
recent coronavirus pandemic has forced most of us to cover up with
masks, making the whole world "smize" at one another to portray our
feelings and reactions through our squinted eyes.

Laughter has long been advocated as the best medicine. Ancient
Greek doctors would send their patients to a "hall of comedians" in the
hospital to help them recover. They practiced "humoural medicine,"
which is based on the premise that the body's balance of fluids, or
"humours" (which means "body fluid" in Latin), controls the balance
between mind and body. The connection between humor, laughter, and
health is even evident in the Bible's Book of Proverbs, which states,
"A cheerful heart is good medicine, but a compressed spirit dries up
the bones." Yet, only in recent years have the numerous psychological
and physical health benefits of a joyful spirit been substantiated by
scientific research.

In the fourteenth century, the prominent medieval French surgeon
Henri de Mondeville began administering humor therapy by reading
jokes to his patients to aid in their healing process after surgery. Several
centuries later, de Mondeville's pioneering use of humor in medicine
was used to treat children by bringing clowns into the hospital, based
on the belief that laughter promotes recuperative effects. In 1979, Dr.
Norman Cousins published a book documenting the effectiveness
of laughter in managing his own chronic pain, after discovering that
"ten minutes of genuine belly laughter caused an anesthetic effect
that would provide at least two hours of pain-free sleep." Cousins'
biochemical research on human emotions was revolutionary in how
it identified the physical benefits of a positive outlook and robust love
of life.

Recent scientific studies show that laughing releases and raises the levels of endorphins, reduces pain, and improves oxygen flow to the heart, brain, and all other organs. Other new research shows that laughing lowers blood pressure, reduces stress hormone levels, boosts immunity, and improves sleep, memory, learning, and performance.

Laughter is a great workout for your respiratory, cardiovascular, and musculoskeletal systems. A deep-rooted belly laugh exercises the diaphragm for improved lung capacity while engaging all of the circumferential trunk musculature. EMG (Electromyographic) tests that examine the electrical activity of your muscles and nerves reveal that all of the core muscles are activated during laughter, especially the obliques (your side abdominal muscles), hence the term "side-splitting laugh."

Smiling and laughing naturally trigger the production of dopamine, which induces a calming effect while promoting pleasure, energy, and motivation. When you feel tense, smile to elicit this mind-body response, or simply relax your jaw muscles by placing your tongue lightly behind your upper teeth. Even when life is stressful and you may not feel like smiling, fake it until you make it better! Approach everything you do with playfulness and delight for a more joyful experience, whether it's meditation, exercise, or work. Smile from the inside out and get your giggle on to make all activities more enjoyable and core-empowering. Laugh your core into optimal holistic health and wellness!

Nature

"The answer, my friend, is blowing in the wind."
—Bob Dylan

In case you needed another reason to go off-screen and on-green more often, spending time outdoors actually empowers your core, in addition to many other key benefits. Studies show exercising outdoors is more beneficial than exercising indoors, both psychologically and physically. Outdoor activities correlate with longer life spans and fewer health problems, such as obesity, depression, asthma, anxiety, mood disorders, high blood pressure, vision problems, heart problems, and chronic pain. People who exercise outdoors, whether at beaches, forests, parks, or gardens, are more likely to stick to their goals and practice regularly.

Spending time in the serenity of nature awakens your senses and promotes clarity, positive thinking, improved coping skills, resilience, and nourishment for your body and spirit through vitamin D and the sense of awe that recent research has shown is important for optimal health and happiness. This sense of awe is attributed by some to mysterious quantum philosophical properties of universal energy, while others find in nature a spiritual connection to a higher deity. As Einstein wrote, "He who can no longer pause to wonder and stand rapt in awe, is as good as dead; his eyes are closed."

I was first introduced to this concept as a young girl summering with my siblings and cousins at our family cabin in the scenic splendor of the Niagara Escarpment in Canada, a steep rock face still blessed with rivers and waterfalls of the ancient sea that once extended from Rochester, New York to Sault Sainte Marie, Ontario. It had been a long day of outdoor adventures, and all of us were exhausted but excited to stay up later than usual, as our parents were all still singing and laughing inside. I remember listening by firelight to my older cousin, Adrian Ivakhiv, as he discussed theories regarding the power of nature and its influence on people. I listened intently with intrigue to his ideas regarding Earth's natural energy, which he has developed in his research and teachings as a professor of environmental philosophy and director of the EcoCultureLab at the University of Vermont, where he continues to study the fascinating connection between environmental energy and the human body.

From an evolutionary perspective, our deep, organic, and visceral connection with nature is intuitive, as humans have been evolving in the natural world for more than two million years. Our lengthy relationship with Mother Earth and all her wonders (flora and fauna) has fostered "biophilia," or our innate need to bond with nature. Our connection to the wonders of nature, and the importance of this connection for optimal health, have a long history in philosophy, religion, art, and culture, yet it has only recently been recognized and validated by the scientific world.

There is abundant evidence that our affiliation with animals, plants, landscapes, and wilderness enhances our holistic health in mind-body-spirit, and is valuable for our journey to core empowerment. Hiking, running, cycling, mountain biking, snowboarding, skiing, paddle boarding, and surfing are all excellent, empowering activities that allow you to challenge your core and harness the energy of nature.

"A ship is always safe at shore, but that is not what it's built for."
—Albert Einstein

Variable terrain, grueling climbs, and sketchy descents along nature trails demand extra agility and responsiveness from your core while hiking or trail running. Cycling is another great core-empowering activity that is gentler on your back, hips, knees, and ankles. As a beginner, cycling indoors, on the road, or on a path builds the foundation for core stability by developing your postural control. Once you've established a solid core foundation, explore mountain biking (or off-road biking) to navigate hills and rough terrain that will kick your core into gear.

Hit the slopes or the surf to center yourself. Snowboarding and skiing are unique core activators, as they lock in your base of support while challenging your core at high velocities. Skiing is easier to learn, yet harder to master, while snowboarding is more difficult to learn, yet easier to master. Paddle-boarding is another comprehensive and empowering outdoor activity, as it engages your core through muscle activation from your fingers to your toes, while forcing you to maintain postural control on an unstable surface and connect to the rhythmic energy of the tidal ebbs and flows. Surfing is debatably the most core-empowering activity of all, as you must constantly adjust your core to balance on a board propelled on an ever-changing surface, adapting to every wave as a new creation of the reach and retreat of the ocean.

I have found that maintaining awareness of my core while doing all of these empowering activities enhances my balance, control, reaction time, and overall skill, while encouraging core control with a low center of gravity. All of these outdoor activities challenge and empower the core in novel ways, and provide physiological, psychological, and spiritual benefits that connect us with nature. So, head outdoors to exercise your core and reconnect with what it means to be human. Following your own passions and unique gifts will give you purpose as you illuminate and empower your core. Find what floats your boat and enjoy the journey!

Core-Empowering Strategies for Kids

"Play gives children a chance to practice what they are learning."
—Fred Rogers

Exercise has an extraordinary capacity to develop a strong body, mind, and spirit in children. This protects them from stress, depression, illness, and symptoms of autism and attention deficit disorders, while improving academic performance and overall happiness. Young children have an amazing capacity for joy, adventure, and presence in the moment. As kids grow older, this capacity must be nurtured to counteract the stresses of life, school, technology, and potential injuries.

Once you equate the amount of training and therefore the subsequent skill obtained, injury rates between girls and boys become more similar. In sports such as downhill skiing, gymnastics, and dance, in which girls begin core training and learn to center themselves at a younger age, disparities in injury rates decline. The differences in female injury rates are not present because girls are incapable, nor are they inherent in their sex; the differences exist because girls haven't been trained to move well. Strength, flexibility, endurance, balance, physical and emotional resilience, nutrition, and life choices are all fully modifiable, and the rate and magnitude of improvements from training in all of these areas is similar in males and females. Resilience to injury is not an inborn trait; it must be nurtured and acquired.

Training the core for stability and movement should begin during infancy and continue throughout one's lifetime. Early training can be initiated by challenging little girls and boys with fun activities to develop core awareness and control with tummy time, bouncing, balancing, swinging, and other forms of physical play. Encourage children to fly like a bird on their bellies, lifting the arms, chest, and legs off the ground. This is a great way to counteract all the flexing and bending activities kids do, and work the muscles that extend the trunk backwards. This helps prevent the common anterior/posterior chain imbalances that compromise core stability.

The best way for children to develop core stability is through fun, outdoor play that incorporates running, jumping, climbing, or just exploring and searching for animals, all of which awaken the senses. Most children today need encouragement to unplug from technology and get moving. Participation in sports provides children with the joy of play and an opportunity for physical and mental development.

Engaging in athletic activities will improve a child's strength, endurance, core stability, and overall health. Nurture a love for adventure and nature by hiking and cycling with baby carriers when they are young, progressing to tandem and independent cycling as children grow up. Make the exercise more exciting by thinking of a creative name to call it other than "exercise," which seems more like a chore to a child. Get kids outside. Let them use their imagination and creativity to have fun while learning to move in new and challenging ways. Every child has the potential to become a great athlete, but those who are regularly allowed to run, play, and try new movements will have a much greater advantage because of all the extra practice moving their bodies.

Let kids empower their cores with fun games like tug of war, wheelbarrow races, trampoline jumping, skating, swimming, swinging, or creative obstacle courses that allow them to walk, crawl, and slither. When my son was younger, we loved playing dinosaur—we would chase each other on the beach pretending to be Velociraptors, Pterodactyls, and T-Rexes. As John Muir once said, "The power of imagination makes us infinite."

Such creative and complex activities enhance mental and physical well-being not only by providing the foundation for all gross and fine motor tasks of daily living, but also by improving posture and core stability, which prevents future musculoskeletal problems throughout the rest of their lives. Posture has a powerful influence on the way children feel and the way they are perceived. Encourage awareness and confidence in children by asking them to explore how they feel when they strike a power pose and imitate their favorite superhero or monster.

It's not so easy for young kids to understand how to activate their core muscles because they have to learn through experience, but a good trick is to ask them to tighten their tummy muscles as if they were going to get a punch in their belly. If you lightly tap the sides of their waist with your fist, instead of near their navel, they will learn to activate all the muscles of the trunk that act in unison like a corset for 360 degrees of stabilization, rather than just the front abdominal muscles (and you'll usually elicit a chuckle).

Explain to your child that these are the muscles that are important to throw a ball, climb a tree, play sports better, and build a base from which they can explore and experience the world in a safer way without injury. The earlier in life that you start training the core, the better—but it's never too late to start. When children learn to train their cores, they will feel better, gain the confidence to try new activities with less fear of hurting themselves, and achieve a boost in their athletic performance.

As parents, we are filled with love, admiration, and fear each time our children climb trees or play in potentially dangerous ways. I recognize the challenge of negotiating the razor thin edge between being overprotective and encouraging your child to be brave, explore the world, and challenge their core. Excessive fear of injury takes away the joy of living. Allow nature to nurture a child's backbone (literally and figuratively) for a strong and resilient core!

Seeds for Thought

- Which activities do you plan to try to further develop your core?

- Have you noticed how laughter engages your core and induces a calming effect while promoting pleasure, energy, and motivation?

- What are some of your favorite outdoor activities?

- Can you think of more ways to connect with nature in your daily life?

- Of all the core empowering activities discussed, which one stirs your passion to empower your core?

CHAPTER 13

Personalize Your Core BASE

"Doctors won't make you healthy. Nutritionists won't make you
slim. Teachers won't make you smart. Gurus won't make you calm.
Mentors won't make you rich. Trainers won't make you fit. Ultimately
you have to take responsibility."
—Naval Ravikant

You are unique! Your core and your journey should be just as unique as you are. Over the years, I have learned from my patients that one size does not fit all. Therefore, prescribing an exercise program that suits the needs and goals of every person is no simple task. I am providing written and video instructions for a beginner "chill" workout and an advanced "intense" workout that may be performed three times per week, but it is imperative that you listen to your own body to determine what is right for you at the moment.

When performing the exercises from the Core BASE Guide, focus on your breath and the quality of your movements, rather than the quantity. Do not feel pressured to complete all the repetitions suggested, as it is more important to maintain good form. Be patient and do not judge yourself when you make a mistake or fail to live up to your expectations. Be grateful for the progress you make, and continue practicing. You will see significant improvements over time if you stick with it.

The house built on sand is swept away by the rain, flood, and winds, whereas the house built on rock withstands the deleterious forces of nature. This parable, found in the New Testament, poignantly describes the importance of a solid and stable foundation. Dig deep and find the foundation of your own core to prepare you for all adversity, sustain your health and wellness through all your endeavors, and build the home of your dreams for your mind-body-spirit.

Chill Core Workout

> "Better to light a candle than to curse the darkness."
> —Chinese Proverb

Breathe

- Complete the Core-Empowering Stretches (listed below and illustrated in Table 1).

- Complete one repetition of each stretch for one minute, focusing on the power of your breath.

- For the first 30 seconds, warm your core up by moving through the three phases, then hold a static sustained stretch at your comfortable end range of motion for 30 seconds, for a total duration of at least 60 seconds.

Awaken and Grow
Core Butterfly
Trunk Twist (with feet on ground)
Dynamic Cat (sitting or standing if unable to go on hands and knees)
Dynamic Dog (with hands on chair)
Heart Opener (with strap or belt)
Tree in the Wind

Awareness

- Complete the Core Awareness Exercises (listed below and illustrated in Table 2).

- Complete 1–2 sets of 7–12 repetitions of each exercise. Hold each repetition for at least 5 seconds.

- Rest one minute between sets, using this time to truly let go of tension and relax with meditation strategies of FAM, OMM, and TM.

Bug (alternate arm and leg lifts)
Bridge
Modified Bird Dog (with pillow or cushion)
Plank (on forearms and/or bent knees)
Side Plank (on forearm and/or bent knees)
Shallow squats
Modified Warrior

Stability

Choose 3 exercises from the following, and complete 1–2 sets of 7–12 repetitions of each exercise:

The Core Balance Exercises (Table 3)
Core Med Ball Exercises (Table 4, using 0–2-pound weights)

Empowerment

Choose at least 3 daily core-empowering activities:

Pilates
Yoga
Martial Arts
Dance
Music
Laughter
Nature

You can find free video demonstrations of each of these exercises at doczaz.com.

Intense Core Workout

"No pressure, no diamonds."
—Thomas Carlyle

Breathe

- Complete the Core-Empowering Stretches (listed below and illustrated in Table 1).
- Complete one repetition of each stretch and hold for one minute each, focusing on the power of your breath.
- For the first 30 seconds, warm your core up by moving through the three phases, then hold a static sustained stretch at your comfortable end range of motion for 30 seconds, for a total duration of at least 60 seconds.

Awaken and Grow
Core Butterfly
Trunk Twist
Dynamic Cat
Dynamic Dog
Heart Opener
Tree in the Wind

Awareness

- Complete the Core Awareness Exercises (listed below and illustrated in Table 2).
- Perform 3 sets of 7–12 repetitions for 5 seconds each to develop strength.
- Cycle through the Awareness exercises as a circuit without rest.
- Work your way up to holding each pose for 30 seconds or more by the end of the third set to develop endurance of the core muscles.
- As you maintain your posture, fortify your mind-core connection with meditation strategies of FAM, OMM and TM.

Bug with crazy limbs
Bridge with alternate leg lifts
Bird Dog with limb motion
Plank on hands with shoulder taps
Side Plank on one hand with starfish pose
Single-Leg Squat
Warrior with limb motion

Stability

Choose 3 exercises from the following, and complete 3 sets of 7–12 repetitions of each exercise:

The Core-Empowering Dynamic Balance Exercises (Table 3)
The Core Med Ball Exercises (Table 4, use minimum 3-pound weights)
The Core-Stabilizing Exercises (Table 5)
The Core Plyometric Exercises (Table 6)
The Core Suspension Exercises (Table 7)

Empowerment

Choose at least 3 daily empowering activities:

Pilates
Yoga
Martial Arts
Dance
Song
Laughter
Nature

You can find free video demonstrations for each of the exercises at doczaz.com.

Your Core Score

"Challenge yourself; it's the only path which leads to growth."
—Morgan Freeman

You may have heard endurance athletes refer to their "PR," or personal record, which refers to their best time in a race of a specific distance. A challenging goal keeps you inspired, as competing against yourself is a great motivator. To assess your own core stability, the Core Score will help you measure your progress. This assessment tool incorporates the most relevant clinical evaluations that correlate with validated laboratory core stability tests. Each posture must be maintained with good form for 30 seconds to score a point, with 21 total possible points (Table 8). I like to have my patients score themselves based on their breath cycles instead of time in order to improve awareness, with a point scored for three slow, deep breaths (full inhalations and exhalations).

Begin with the Bridge of the Awareness exercises for one point, extending one leg straight while balancing on your other leg for two points, and raising the heel of your weightbearing leg for three points. Begin the side-plank test on your forearm for one point, on your hand for two points, and raise your non-weightbearing arm and leg toward the sky for three points. For the standard plank, one point is earned on your forearms, two points on your hands, and three points if you can lift each hand to the opposite shoulder. Stay on your belly now for the Cobra and lift your chest off the ground with your hands at your sides for one point, hands at your ears for two points, and hands overhead like a superhero for three points.

Next, get on your hands and knees in the quadruped position and push up with your toes to slightly lift your knees off the ground (1-2 inches) for a Floating Cat to score one point. Lift one foot slightly off the ground for two points, and try lifting the opposite hand so you are balancing on one foot and the opposite hand before switching for three points. The Y balance test challenges how far you can reach with your foot in all three directions of a Y formation, just as in the Y Balance Stabilizing exercise. Reach your foot in each direction: one foot-length for one point, two foot-lengths for two points, and three foot-lengths for three points. And finally, squat down to about

45 degrees at your knees for one point (a shallow squat), 90 degrees (like sitting in a chair) for two points, and a shallow squat on one leg (45 degrees) for three points. Be sure to check your form in a mirror, if possible, to avoid leaning with your trunk or collapsing your knees inward.

If you achieve a perfect Core Score of 21, congratulations! Just remember to set your goals just beyond your current reach to always have something to strive for. Raise the bar of your own Core Score as I do with high-level athletes. For example, athletes may set their squat goals at 90 degrees for one point, a shallow squat on one leg (45 degrees) for two points, and a 90-degree single leg squat for 3 points. Celebrate your achievements, then dig deeper and raise the bar a little higher each time you succeed!

Go to doczaz.com for free video demonstrations.

Table 8. The Core Score

Core test	1 Point	2 Points	3 Points	Core Score
Bridge				
Side Plank				
Prone Plank (Push Up Position)				
Cobra (On belly raising chest off ground)				
Floating Cat (In quadruped position holding knees slightly off ground)				
Y Balance (Standing on one leg and reaching with the other foot in Y position)				
Squat				
Total				

Conclusion

The Future of Core Empowerment

"The moment we decide to fulfill something, we can do anything."
—Greta Thunberg

In 2010, I visited my parents' homeland for the first time. Although we had never met or even spoken, I was lovingly welcomed by my Ukrainian relatives, whose tables were covered with traditional foods and superb homemade wines, which we shared over heart-wrenching stories of my parents' childhoods. My relatives seemed to already know me just from the letters my parents had written to them over the years (the ones that hadn't been intercepted by the corrupt Ukrainian mail system).

As I walked through the small villages, I felt as though I had stepped back in time. Few people had phones, only one person (my cousin) had a car, and not one home had indoor plumbing. They lived simple lives, but were generous, loving, and had a deep sense of community. Since that visit, technology has significantly improved, with my distant family now readily accessible through the internet and social media.

Like my family in Ukraine, people who were once isolated in remote areas everywhere now have the world at their fingertips, uniting us all under one sky. This expansion of community, or gathering of worldwide spirit, has the potential for boundless change. Technological globalization holds great promise for the future of health and wellness, as well as equality regardless of sex, race, or socio-economic status.

The recent global health emergency of the novel coronavirus pandemic has accelerated technological changes that will change healthcare indefinitely throughout the world. The growth of telehealth (the provision of healthcare by the remote means of telecommunications) and other electronic platforms of healthcare delivery have been catalyzed out of need, and will have a durable impact on the way we practice medicine in the future. Access to services has improved on a tremendous scale, yet we also recognize that disparities in access persist, requiring focused and ongoing efforts. International attention is now focused on the viability of leveraging telehealth to democratize medical expertise across communities around the globe. There is despair, hardship, and adversity throughout the world, but these shared challenges promote collaboration, and collaboration fortifies the collective consciousness of the international community. A strong, unified community inspires change to promote wellness for all.

The evolving technology of telehealth has limitless potential to generate change by reaching and empowering people all over the world through education regarding core health and wellness. My experience in developing the telehealth program at Yale provides an optimistic vision for the future of core health thanks to this revolutionary virtual technology. The success of virtual exercise, which combines avatar coaching, 3D motion-capture technology, and remote clinical oversight, has been demonstrated in our newly published research.

Lifestyle medicine and wellness practitioners will be able to utilize technology to move forward for the next generation of health promotion. Our findings support the effectiveness, benefits, and potential of telehealth to provide optimal wellness and empowerment so all can achieve the fullness of life, vitality, and flourishing that characterizes a high level of well-being.

"Let us make our future now, and let us make our dreams tomorrow's reality."
—Malala Yousafzai

Futurists predict the world will continue evolving to a techno-driven state of oneness, where artificial intelligence and humans work in harmony. Predictions for the future include contact lenses that will move objects with mind power, tiny robots that can be injected into our bloodstream to cure diseases, and rocket taxis that will zoom us off to other planets. Such speculations are difficult to imagine, as are the advances of each generation to the prior.

I doubt that either of my grandmothers, born in the 1890s, envisioned their granddaughter finishing an Ironman Triathlon, becoming a doctor, or devoting her career to women's health research. Feminism in Ukraine was considered counterrevolutionary until the fall of the Soviet regime in the 1990s. Since then, women's rights groups have evolved to fight for equality in terms of how women are perceived, promoted, and valued, but these groups are still subject to intimidation from the government. Women worldwide face these same challenges, which not only affect them politically and professionally, but also physically, psychologically, and emotionally.

The science that informs medicine and health (including prevention, diagnosis, and treatment) has historically failed to consider the crucial effect of one's sex. Significant progress to resolve inequality has been made since 1993, when the National Institute of Health mandated that women be included in any government-funded health research. Over the past four decades, male and female international researchers have united in solidarity to make great strides in our understanding of neuromuscular differences between the sexes in core stability, and how effective strategies can be applied to reduce injuries.

Lifestyle medicine, health promotion, and core wellness will continue to play critical roles in health and quality of life. Through universal collaboration of diversity-infused research and widespread education, we will improve the future of health, and level the playing field for all races, sexes, and socio-economic statuses when it comes to injury prevention.

My three decades in the medical field have taught me a tremendous amount about the impact and manifestation of injury, how to help injured patients find their way back to the lives they envisioned, and how to prevent these traumatic events from occurring in the first place. This invaluable clinical experience, together with my health and injury prevention research, has been systematized into this integrated, holistic Core BASE Guide to harness the power of your mind-body-spirit.

You have learned how The Core BASE employs an easily tailored, comprehensive action plan to establish a solid mind-core connection, transform your body, fortify your relationship with self-care and exercise, and nurture, nourish, and empower your core for a healthful, happy life. The term "core stability" has been commercialized and misconstrued, leading unwitting victims astray with endless sit-ups and swinging kettlebells, and onto a fast track to injury and despair. This book highlights how the core is much more than "six-pack abs," but rather a powerhouse of physical, emotional, and spiritual flourishing.

Now you understand what core stability truly means from a scientific perspective, and how a stable core directly is necessary to reduce injury rates in both women and men. Although females are more vulnerable to problems in their bones and joints, that is not to say that women are unequal to men, or that we need to make women's bodies behave more like men's. We ask girls to "bend it like Beckham," yet the female body is not built, nor does it function, like Beckham's. This book does not attempt to turn girls into boys, or women into men, but aims to highlight sex-based differences to optimize every body's full power potential for daily life activities and sports.

The Core BASE Guide has taught you how to train your core through a guided progression of Breathing, Awareness, Stability, and Empowerment, beginning with the inner core toner exercise and progressing through seven tables of seven core exercises to build your BASE. You have learned to develop your core foundation with the essential building block of your inner core squad in the Breathing Phase, fortified this foundation with the whole core team in the Awareness Phase, integrated the team with your whole body's kinetic chain in the Stability Phase, and enlightened your core to unleash your full mind-body-spirit potential in the Empowerment Phase.

With the Core BASE, you now have all the tools, strategies, and techniques you need to establish your mind-core oneness. This will allow you to tune in to your core to improve your body image for a leaner, trimmer, stronger, more powerful, healthy, and happy core with the following lessons for empowerment:

- Strategies for meditation and healthy breathing for optimal inner core activation.

- Tips for improving posture, which will slim down and trim your figure, improve the fit of your clothing, ease the stress of computer work, and reduce your risk of future injuries, aches, and pains.

- Techniques for improving your core resiliency, with improved strength, flexibility, and efficiency of movement for everyday activities, such as bending, turning, reaching, lifting, gardening, or performing work-related tasks while sitting or standing for prolonged periods.

- Methods for developing a strong foundation of power for activities that you currently enjoy or would love to try, such as marathons, racket sports, golf, kayaking, surfing, cycling, snowboarding, rock climbing, or your favorite exercise or dance class with improved confidence and decreased risk of harm.

- Tips for improving your bone health and life longevity, reducing your stress, enhancing your sexuality, and improving your positive outlook and quality of life.

Whether you are hoping to develop the body image you always wanted, uncover the secret to living a healthier life without injury, or just feel better, you will benefit from the Core BASE Guide. It is imperative that the invaluable information of this guide be accessible to all, to establish widespread implementation for the empowerment of all in mind, body, and soul. Embark on this groundbreaking step-by-step journey to holistic wellness to get to the "core" of your magnificent self and harness your incredible power from within!

Gratitude

I am deeply grateful to my family, friends, colleagues, co-investigators, patients, and students for their wonderful support and invaluable contributions to the integration and grounding of The Core BASE.

Glossary

ACL Anterior Cruciate Ligament: A tissue in the knee that connects the thigh bone with the shin bone. This ligament is often implicated in serious knee injuries, and often occurs from a non-contact injury mechanism, such as landing, cutting, pivoting, or twisting.

Amortization phase: The very brief moment in a jump when a muscle rebounds to generate explosive power.

Biomechanics: The study of the structure, function, and motion of the mechanical aspects of the body's team, with the core as the most valuable player.

Center of gravity (center of mass): The point of the body at which weight is evenly dispersed and all sides are in balance.

Closed Kinetic Chain: The state of the body segments when the hand/hands or foot/feet are fixed with constant contact to an immobile surface, with multiple segments of the body contracting at the same time to stabilize and control movements across multiple joints. Closed chain exercises, such as push-ups, pull-ups, squats, leg presses, and lunges are more functional because they train your muscles in ways that mimic the movements performed in real life and sports.

Core: The body's center of balance and strength. Includes 35 muscles (abdominal, back, pelvic, and glutes), the spine, and hip joints.

Core stability: Trunk control that allows production, transfer, and control of force and motion from the anatomical center to all parts of the body. It is the ability to set the body in motion and control the body throughout this motion.

Crepitus: Harmless grinding, creaking, crunching, and/or popping in your joints, without the presence of pain.

Diaphragmatic breathing (belly breathing): Deep, healthy breathing that maximally expands the lungs and abdomen to optimally engage the core muscles and promote the health of mind-body-spirit.

Distal: Situated farther away from the center of the body in relation to another part.

Delayed Onset Muscle Soreness (DOMS): Normal discomfort and stiffness felt in muscles several hours or days after unaccustomed or strenuous exercise.

Epigenetics: The field of research that examines how our daily choices (psychological outlook, diet, exercise, and other lifestyle choices) influence the way our genes are expressed in our bodies and those of our offspring to improve our ability to fight disease, prevent injury, and promote overall wellbeing.

Focused Attention Meditation (FAM): The practice of connecting your mind to your inner core by tuning in to your breathing and inner core activation to increase brain power and connectivity, while establishing the foundation of core stability.

Global Core Muscles: The large, outer muscles of the trunk and pelvis that produce high forces and large movements, indirectly affecting the vertebrae and supporting them as the prime movers. These powerful muscles get all the glory for a sculpted physique.

Hook Lying Position: A position that entails lying on your back with knees bent and feet flat on the ground, and with your spine in its neutral, natural alignment.

Holistic: Comprehensive of all the parts of the whole person, considering body, mind, and spirit.

Kinetic Chain: The system by which all of the muscles, bones, and joints work together as interconnected segments of the body to function optimally, with the core as the central, most powerful link.

Local Core Muscles: The deeper, inner stabilizing muscles of the trunk and pelvis that control individual vertebral segments with precision. These deep muscles quietly activate behind the scenes to anticipate your next move and activate appropriately to support you, fine-tune your movement, and save you from injury.

Mantra: From Sanskrit, an "instrument of thought" that facilitates transcendence to new levels of core awareness and optimal core empowerment.

Meditation: The practice of tuning out the external and getting in tune with your internal universe for core awareness and empowerment. See also Focused Attention Meditation, Open Monitoring Meditation, and Transcendental Meditation.

Natural Spine: The shape of a neutral spinal alignment with three curves, which is the optimal position for core stability.

Neuromuscular control: The ability to coherently engage all of the trunk muscles in harmony to achieve core stability with precise timing, strength, coordination, and endurance at the right time, for the correct duration, and with the right combination of forces to control, direct, and maximize all the movements of your body for efficiency and effectiveness.

Open Kinetic Chain: The state of the body's chain of segments when the hand/hands or foot/feet are free in space, not on a surface such as the ground, the wall, a tabletop, or the platform of a weight machine. Examples of an open chain activity include waving your hand or lifting your leg. Open chain exercises are great for improving strength and function in isolation.

Open Monitoring Meditation (OMM): The practice of observation or nonreactive monitoring of the core without judgement, by simply perceiving and developing awareness of breath, posture, and core function through the natural stream of consciousness.

Pandiculation: Nature's way of aligning your core by moving back and forth between extreme positions of the spine to reset your body's software and reboot your sensation and control of your muscles to their optimal functioning length to release muscular and emotional tension, reduce pain, increase mobility, improve your posture, and align your trunk for optimal performance.

Perturbation: A challenge to the balance of the body's center.

Plyometrics: Jump training that develops core stability and ability to generate power in everything you do. In these exercises, your muscles actively stretch before immediately shortening. The faster this transition occurs, the more power is generated, and the higher you can jump.

Proprioception: The ability to perceive position and movement of each part of the body. This perception, or awareness, is obtained from sensors in your joints and muscles, and relayed to and from the brain through the nerves. This information is then used by the brain to generate appropriate control to the core muscles to make the proper adjustments so you can move your body in an optimal manner.

Proximal: Situated closer to the center of the body in relation to another part.

Quadruped: A position with hands and knees on the ground, with hands placed directly under the shoulders and knees directly under the hips.

Transcendental Meditation (TM): A strategy for developing self-realization and a higher state of consciousness which reduces distraction, stress, anxiety, blood pressure, and overall cardiovascular health, while improving clarity, focus, brain functioning, creativity, energy, and awareness of the core.

Vagus Nerve: The longest "wandering" nerve in your body that connects your brain to many important organs throughout the body, traveling from your head to your chest and abdomen, and branching out to the gut, heart, and lungs. This critical nerve is also a key part of your parasympathetic nervous system.

Vestibular System: A sensory system of the inner ear that acts as a carpenter's level for the body, contributing to the sense of balance and spatial orientation for coordinated movement.

About the Author

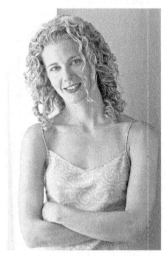

Photograph © Benjamin Dimmitt

Bohdanna "Billie" Zazulak DPT, OCS is the principal investigator and author of the first published research to establish a scientific link between core stability and reduced injury rates. Dr. Zazulak won the highly regarded and prestigious Rose Award from the American Physical Therapy Association for her groundbreaking research, and has three decades of experience as an American Physical Therapy Association Orthopedic Certified Specialist, a Doctor of Physical Therapy in Sports Medicine and Orthopedics, and a researcher and faculty member at Yale New Haven Hospital and Yale University School of Medicine. Dr. Zazulak's pioneering research on core stability, injury prevention, and rehabilitation has been published in top-tier medical journals and textbooks in medical and physical therapy curricula. Her main interest is in promoting core stability for all women and men so that fewer injuries will occur in their younger lives, and fewer incapacities will be experienced in their older adult lives. Dr. Zazulak received her Bachelor of Science in Physical Therapy from the State University of New York, Master of Science in Orthopedic Physical Therapy from Quinnipiac University, and Doctorate of Physical Therapy from Temple University, and now works and lives in Connecticut, where she was recently recognized as a "Top Doctor" in the region by Women in Medicine.

References

Acevedo, Bianca P., Sarah Pospos, and Helen Lavretsky. "The Neural Mechanisms of Meditative Practices: Novel Approaches for Healthy Aging." Current Behavioral Neuroscience Reports 3, no. 4 (2016): 328–39. https://doi.org/10.1007/s40473-016-0098-x.

Aguilera-Castells, Joan, Bernat Buscà, Azahara Fort-Vanmeerhaeghe, Alicia M. Montalvo, and Javier Peña. "Muscle activation in suspension training: a systematic review." Sports Biomechanics 14 (2018):1-21. https://doi.org/10.1080/14763141.2018.1472293.

Aljuraifani, Rafeef, Ryan E. Stafford, Leanne M. Hall, Wolbert van den Hoorn, and Paul W. Hodges. "Task-Specific Differences in Respiration-Related Activation of Deep and Superficial Pelvic Floor Muscles." Journal of Applied Physiology (1985) 126, no. 5 (2019): 1343–51. https://doi.org/10.1152/japplphysiol.00704.2018.

Almousa, S., H. Moser, G. Kitsoulis, N. Almousa, H. Tzovaras, and D. Kastani. "The Prevalence of Urine Incontinence in Nulliparous Female Athletes: a Systematic Review." Physiotherapy 101 (2015). https://doi.org/10.1016/j.physio.2015.03.178.

AlQatari, Abdullah A, Jawad A. Alturki, Komail A. Abdulali, Dawood A. Alhumud, Mohammed A. Alibrahim, Yaser A. Alarab, Ayad M. Salem, et al. "Changes in Heart Rate Variability and Baroreflex Sensitivity During Daytime Naps." Nature and Science of Sleep Volume 12 (2020): 661–69. https://doi.org/10.2147/nss.s270191.

Aoki, Yoshitaka, Heidi W. Brown, Linda Brubaker, Jean Nicolas Cornu, J. Oliver Daly, and Rufus Cartwright. "Urinary Incontinence in Women." Nature Reviews Disease Primers 3, no. 1 (2017). https://doi.org/10.1038/nrdp.2017.42.

Arida, Ricardo Mario, and Lavinia Teixeira-Machado. "The Contribution of Physical Exercise to Brain Resilience." Frontiers in Behavioral Neuroscience 14 (2021). https://doi.org/10.3389/fnbeh.2020.626769.

Basso, Julia C., Alexandra McHale, Victoria Ende, Douglas J. Oberlin, and Wendy A. Suzuki. "Brief, Daily Meditation Enhances Attention, Memory, Mood, and Emotional Regulation IN Non-Experienced Meditators." Behavioural Brain Research 356 (2019): 208–20. https://doi.org/10.1016/j.bbr.2018.08.023.

Behm, David G., Anthony J. Blazevich, Anthony D. Kay, and Malachy McHugh. "Acute Effects of Muscle Stretching on Physical Performance, Range of Motion, and Injury Incidence in Healthy Active Individuals: a Systematic Review." Applied Physiology, Nutrition, and Metabolism 41, no. 1 (2016): 1–11. https://doi.org/10.1139/apnm-2015-0235.

Ben Ami, Noa, and Gali Dar. "What Is the Most Effective Verbal Instruction for Correctly Contracting the Pelvic Floor Muscles?" Neurourology and Urodynamics 37, no. 8 (2018): 2904–10. https://doi.org/10.1002/nau.23810.

Bertolucci, Luiz Fernando. "Pandiculation: Nature's Way of Maintaining the Functional Integrity of the Myofascial System?" Journal of Bodywork and Movement Therapies 15, no. 3 (2011): 268–80. https://doi.org/10.1016/j.jbmt.2010.12.006.

Biscarini, Andrea, Samuele Contemori, and Giuditta Grolla. "Activation of Scapular and Lumbopelvic Muscles During Core Exercises Executed on a Whole-Body Wobble Board." Journal of Sport Rehabilitation 28, no. 6 (2019): 623–34. https://doi.org/10.1123/jsr.2018-0089.

Bjerkefors, Anna, Maria M. Ekblom, Karin Josefsson, and Alf Thorstensson. "Deep and Superficial Abdominal Muscle Activation during Trunk Stabilization Exercises with and without Instruction to Hollow." Manual Therapy 15, no. 5 (2010): 502–7. https://doi.org/10.1016/j.math.2010.05.006.

Bø, Kari, and Ingrid Elisabeth Nygaard. "Is Physical Activity Good or Bad for the Female Pelvic Floor? A Narrative Review." Sports Medicine 50, no. 3 (2019): 471–84. https://doi.org/10.1007/s40279-019-01243-1.

Boccia, Maddalena, Laura Piccardi, and Paola Guariglia. "The Meditative Mind: A Comprehensive Meta-Analysis of MRI

Studies." BioMed Research International (2015): 419808. https://doi.org/10.1155/2015/419808.

Bordoni, Bruno, and Emiliano Zanier. "Anatomic Connections of the Diaphragm Influence of Respiration on the Body System." Journal of Multidisciplinary Healthcare, 2013, 281. https://doi.org/10.2147/jmdh.s45443.

Bradley, Helen and Joseph Esformes. "Breathing pattern disorders and functional movement." International Journal of Sports Physical Therapy, 2014, 9(1): 28-39. PubMed Central.

Brennan L, de Roos B. Nutrigenomics: lessons learned and future perspectives. Am J Clin Nutr. 2021 Mar 11;113(3):503-516. https://doi.org/10.1093/ajcn/nqaa366.

Butler, Cody R., Kirsten Allen, Lindsay J. DiStefano, and Lindsey K. Lepley. "Protracted Cardiovascular Impairments After Anterior Cruciate Ligament Injury: A Critically Appraised Topic." Journal of Sport Rehabilitation 29, no. 5 (2019): 680–83. https://doi.org/10.1123/jsr.2019-0175.

Calatayud, Joaquin, Jose Casaña, Fernando Martín, Markus D. Jakobsen, Juan C. Colado, Pedro Gargallo, Álvaro Juesas, Víctor Muñoz, and Lars L. Andersen. "Trunk Muscle Activity during Different Variations of the Supine Plank Exercise." Musculoskeletal Science and Practice 28 (2017): 54–58. https://doi.org/10.1016/j.msksp.2017.01.011.

Campanelli, Stephany, Adriano Bretanha Lopes Tort, and Bruno Lobão-Soares. "Pranayamas and Their Neurophysiological Effects." International Journal of Yoga 13, no. 3 (2020): 183. https://doi.org/10.4103/ijoy.ijoy_91_19.

Cannon, Jordan, Edward D.J. Cambridge, and Stuart M. McGill. "Increased Core Stability Is Associated with Reduced Knee Valgus during Single-Leg Landing Tasks: Investigating Lumbar Spine and Hip Joint Rotational Stiffness." Journal of Biomechanics 116 (2021): 110240. https://doi.org/10.1016/j.jbiomech.2021.110240.

Carbone, Andrew, and Scott Rodeo. "Review of Current Understanding of Post-Traumatic Osteoarthritis Resulting from Sports Injuries." Journal of Orthopaedic Research 35, no. 3 (2017): 397–405. https://doi.org/10.1002/jor.23341.

Chaabene, Helmi, David G. Behm, Yassine Negra, and Urs Granacher. "Acute Effects of Static Stretching on Muscle Strength and Power: An Attempt to Clarify Previous Caveats." Frontiers in Physiology 10 (2019). https://doi.org/10.3389/fphys.2019.01468.

Chang, Jingjing, Meng Zhang, Glenn Hitchman, Jiang Qiu, and Yijun Liu. "When You Smile, You Become Happy: Evidence from Resting State Task-Based FMRI." Biological Psychology 103 (2014): 100–106. https://doi.org/10.1016/j.biopsycho.2014.08.003.

Chen, Binglin, Yulin Dong, JiaBao Guo, YiLi Zheng, Juan Zhang, and Xueqiang Wang. "Effects of Whole-Body Vibration on Lumbar-Abdominal Muscles Activation in Healthy Young Adults: A Pilot Study." Medical Science Monitor 25 (2019): 1945–51. https://doi.org/10.12659/msm.912720.

Cho, Misuk. "The Effects of Bridge Exercise with the Abdominal Drawing-in Maneuver on an Unstable Surface on the Abdominal Muscle Thickness of Healthy Adults." Journal of Physical Therapy Science 27, no. 1 (2015): 255–57. https://doi.org/10.1589/jpts.27.255.

Cope, Thane, Sarah Wechter, Michaella Stucky, Corey Thomas, and Mark Wilhelm. "The Impact of Lumbopelvic Control on Overhead Performance and Shoulder Injury in Overhead Athletes: A Systematic Review." International Journal of Sports Physical Therapy 14, no. 4 (2019): 500–513. https://doi.org/10.26603/ijspt20190500.

Cortell-Tormo, Juan M., Miguel García-Jaén, Iván Chulvi-Medrano, Sergio Hernández-Sánchez, Ángel G. Lucas-Cuevas, and Juan Tortosa-Martínez. "Influence of Scapular Position on the Core Musculature Activation in the Prone Plank Exercise." Journal of Strength and Conditioning Research 31, no. 8 (2017): 2255–62. https://doi.org/10.1519/jsc.0000000000001689.

Cugliari, Giovanni, and Gennaro Boccia. "Core Muscle Activation in Suspension Training Exercises." Journal of Human Kinetics 56, no. 1 (2017): 61–71. https://doi.org/10.1515/hukin-2017-0023.

Da Silva Borin, Lílian Cristina, Fabiana Roberta Nunes, and Elaine Caldeira de Oliveira Guirro. "Assessment of Pelvic Floor Muscle Pressure in Female Athletes." PM&R 5, no. 3 (2013): 189–93. https://doi.org/10.1016/j.pmrj.2012.09.001.

De Blaiser, Cedric, Roel De Ridder, Tine Willems, Luc Vanden Bossche, Lieven Danneels, and Philip Roosen. "Impaired Core Stability as a Risk Factor for the Development of Lower Extremity Overuse Injuries: A Prospective Cohort Study." The American Journal of Sports Medicine 47, no. 7 (2019): 1713–21. https://doi.org/10.1177/0363546519837724.

De Mattos Lourenco, Thais Regina, Priscila Katsumi Matsuoka, Edmund Chada Baracat, and Jorge Milhem Haddad. "Urinary incontinence in female athletes: a systematic review." International Urogynecology Journal 29, no. 12 (2018): 1757-1763. https://doi.org/10.1007/s00192-018-3629-z.

De Witte, Martina, Ana da Pinho, Geert-Jan Stams, Xavier Moonen, Arjan E.R. Bos, and Susan van Hooren. "Music Therapy for Stress Reduction: a Systematic Review and Meta-Analysis." Health Psychology Review (2020): 1–26. https://doi.org/10.1080/17437199.2020.1846580.

Diekfuss, Jed A., Dustin R. Grooms, Scott Bonnette, Christopher A. DiCesare, Staci Thomas, Ryan P. MacPherson, Jonathan D. Ellis, et al. "Real-Time Biofeedback Integrated into Neuromuscular Training Reduces High-Risk Knee Biomechanics and Increases Functional Brain Connectivity: A Preliminary Longitudinal Investigation." Psychophysiology 57, no. 5 (2020). https://doi.org/10.1111/psyp.13545.

Divine, Jon G, Bohdanna T Zazulak, and Timothy E Hewett. "Viscosupplementation for Knee Osteoarthritis." Clinical Orthopaedics and Related Research 455 (2007): 113–22. https://doi.org/10.1097/blo.0b013e31802f5421.

Ekstrom, Richard A., Robert A. Donatelli, and Kenji C. Carp. "Electromyographic Analysis of Core Trunk, Hip, and Thigh Muscles During 9 Rehabilitation Exercises." Journal of Orthopaedic & Sports Physical Therapy 37, no. 12 (2007): 754–62. https://doi.org/10.2519/jospt.2007.2471.

Ellenbecker, Todd S., and Ryoki Aoki. "Step by Step Guide to Understanding the Kinetic Chain Concept in the Overhead Athlete." Current Reviews in Musculoskeletal Medicine 13, no. 2 (2020): 155–63. https://doi.org/10.1007/s12178-020-09615-1.

El-Sharkawy, Ahmed M., Opinder Sahota, and Dileep N. Lobo. "Acute and Chronic Effects of Hydration Status on Health." Nutrition Reviews 73, no. suppl 2 (2015): 97–109. https://doi.org/10.1093/nutrit/nuv038.

Emerich Gordon, Kate, and Ona Reed. "The Role of the Pelvic Floor in Respiration: A Multidisciplinary Literature Review." Journal of Voice 34, no. 2 (2020): 243–49. https://doi.org/10.1016/j.jvoice.2018.09.024.

Escamilla, Rafael F., Clare Lewis, Amanda Pecson, Rodney Imamura, and James R. Andrews. "Muscle Activation Among Supine, Prone, and Side Position Exercises With and Without a Swiss Ball." Sports Health: A Multidisciplinary Approach 8, no. 4 (2016): 372–79. https://doi.org/10.1177/1941738116653931.

Escamilla, Rafael F., Clare Lewis, Duncan Bell, Gwen Bramblet, Jason Daffron, Steve Lambert, Amanda Pecson, Rodney Imamura, Lonnie Paulos, and James R. Andrews. "Core Muscle Activation During Swiss Ball and Traditional Abdominal Exercises." Journal of Orthopaedic & Sports Physical Therapy 40, no. 5 (2010): 265–76. https://doi.org/10.2519/jospt.2010.3073.

Ferri-Caruana, Ana, Beatriz Prades-Insa, and Pilar Serra-AÑÓ. "Effects of Pelvic and Core Strength Training on Biomechanical Risk Factors for Anterior Cruciate Ligament Injuries." The Journal of Sports Medicine and Physical Fitness 60, no. 8 (2020). https://doi.org/10.23736/s0022-4707.20.10552-8.

Field, Tiffany, Miguel Diego, Maria Hernandez-Reif, Saul Schanberg, Cynthia Kuhn, Regina Yando, and Debra Bendell. "Pregnancy Anxiety and Comorbid Depression and Anger: Effects on the

Fetus and Neonate." Depression and Anxiety 17, no. 3 (2003): 140–51. https://doi.org/10.1002/da.10071.

Findlay, Rebekka J, Eilidh H Macrae, Ian Y Whyte, Chris Easton, and Laura J Forrest (née Whyte). "How the Menstrual Cycle and Menstruation Affect Sporting Performance: Experiences and Perceptions of Elite Female Rugby Players." British Journal of Sports Medicine 54, no. 18 (2020): 1108–13. https://doi.org/10.1136/bjsports-2019-101486.

Foss, Kim D., Staci Thomas, Jane C. Khoury, Gregory D. Myer, and Timothy E. Hewett. "A School-Based Neuromuscular Training Program and Sport-Related Injury Incidence: A Prospective Randomized Controlled Clinical Trial." Journal of Athletic Training 53, no. 1 (2018): 20–28. https://doi.org/10.4085/1062-6050-173-16.

Fultz, Nina E., Giorgio Bonmassar, Kawin Setsompop, Robert A. Stickgold, Bruce R. Rosen, Jonathan R. Polimeni, and Laura D. Lewis. "Coupled Electrophysiological, Hemodynamic, and Cerebrospinal Fluid Oscillations in Human Sleep." Science 366, no. 6465 (2019): 628–31. https://doi.org/10.1126/science.aax5440.

García-Sánchez, E., J.A. Rubio-Arias, V. Ávila-Gandía, D.J. Ramos-Campo, and J. López-Román. "Effectiveness of Pelvic Floor Muscle Training in Treating Urinary Incontinence in Women: A Current Review." Actas Urológicas Españolas (English Edition) 40, no. 5 (2016): 271–78. https://doi.org/10.1016/j.acuroe.2016.03.011.

Garrison, J. Craig, Amanda Arnold, Michael J. Macko, and John E. Conway. "Baseball Players Diagnosed With Ulnar Collateral Ligament Tears Demonstrate Decreased Balance Compared to Healthy Controls." Journal of Orthopaedic & Sports Physical Therapy 43, no. 10 (2013): 752–58. https://doi.org/10.2519/jospt.2013.4680.

GBD 2017 Diet Collaborators. "Health effects of dietary risks in 195 countries, 1990-2017: a systematic analysis for the Global Burden of Disease Study 2017." Lancet 393,10184. (2019):1958-1972. https://doi.org/10.1016/S0140-6736(19)30041-8.

Gerritsen, Roderik J., and Guido P. Band. "Breath of Life: The Respiratory Vagal Stimulation Model of Contemplative Activity." Frontiers in Human Neuroscience 12 (2018). https://doi.org/10.3389/fnhum.2018.00397.

Ghati, Nirmal, Avantika K. Killa, Gautam Sharma, Biju Karunakaran, Aman Agarwal, Sriloy Mohanty, L. Nivethitha, Deepti Siddharthan, and R.M. Pandey. "A Randomized Trial of the Immediate Effect of Bee-Humming Breathing Exercise on Blood Pressure and Heart Rate Variability in Patients with Essential Hypertension." Explore, 2020. https://doi.org/10.1016/j.explore.2020.03.009.

Giagio, Silvia, Stefano Salvioli, Paolo Pillastrini, and Tiziano Innocenti. "Sport and Pelvic Floor Dysfunction in Male and Female Athletes: A Scoping Review." Neurourology and Urodynamics 40, no. 1 (2021): 55–64. https://doi.org/10.1002/nau.24564.

Goyal, Madhav, Sonal Singh, Erica M. Sibinga, Neda F. Gould, Anastasia Rowland-Seymour, Ritu Sharma, Zackary Berger, et al. "Meditation Programs for Psychological Stress and Well-Being." JAMA Internal Medicine 174, no. 3 (2014): 357. https://doi.org/10.1001/jamainternmed.2013.13018.

Greiwe, Justin, Jae Gruenke, and Joanna S. Zeiger. "The Impact of Mental Toughness and Postural Abnormalities on Dysfunctional Breathing in Athletes." Journal of Asthma, 2021, 1–15. https://doi.org/10.1080/02770903.2021.1871739.

Grooms, Dustin R., Jed A. Diekfuss, Jonathan D. Ellis, Weihong Yuan, Jonathan Dudley, Kim D. Foss, Staci Thomas, et al. "A Novel Approach to Evaluate Brain Activation for Lower Extremity Motor Control." Journal of Neuroimaging 29, no. 5 (2019): 580–88. https://doi.org/10.1111/jon.12645.

Hartmann, Dee, and Julie Sarton. "Chronic Pelvic Floor Dysfunction." Best Practice & Research Clinical Obstetrics & Gynaecology 28, no. 7 (2014): 977–90. https://doi.org/10.1016/j.bpobgyn.2014.07.008.

Hauswald, Anne, Teresa Übelacker, Sabine Leske, and Nathan Weisz. "What It Means to Be Zen: Marked Modulations of Local and

Interareal Synchronization during Open Monitoring Meditation." NeuroImage 108 (2015): 265–73. https://doi.org/10.1016/j. neuroimage.2014.12.065.

Hebert, Jeffrey J., Shane L. Koppenhaver, Deydre S. Teyhen, Bruce F. Walker, and Julie M. Fritz. "The Evaluation of Lumbar Multifidus Muscle Function via Palpation: Reliability and Validity of a New Clinical Test." The Spine Journal 15, no. 6 (2015): 1196–1202. https://doi.org/10.1016/j.spinee.2013.08.056.

Heiss, Rafael, Christoph Lutter, Jürgen Freiwald, Matthias Hoppe, Casper Grim, Klaus Poettgen, Raimund Forst, Wilhelm Bloch, Moritz Hüttel, and Thilo Hotfiel. "Advances in Delayed-Onset Muscle Soreness (DOMS) – Part II: Treatment and Prevention." Sportverletzung · Sportschaden 33, no. 01 (2019): 21–29. https:// doi.org/10.1055/a-0810-3516.

Hewett, Timothy E., Stephanie Di Stasi, Gregory Myer. "Current concepts for injury prevention in athletes after anterior cruciate ligament reconstruction." The American Journal of Sports Medicine. (2013): 216-24. https://doi.org/10.1177/0363546512459638.

Hewett, Timothy E., Kevin R. Ford, Yingying Y. Xu, Jane Khoury, and Gregory D. Myer. "Utilization of ACL Injury Biomechanical and Neuromuscular Risk Profile Analysis to Determine the Effectiveness of Neuromuscular Training." The American Journal of Sports Medicine 44, no. 12 (2016): 3146–51. https://doi. org/10.1177/0363546516656373.

Hewett, Timothy E., Kevin R. Ford, Yingying Y. Xu, Jane Khoury, and Gregory D. Myer. "Effectiveness of Neuromuscular Training Based on the Neuromuscular Risk Profile." The American Journal of Sports Medicine 45, no. 9 (2017): 2142–47. https:// doi.org/10.1177/0363546517700128.

Hewett, Timothy E., T. R. Lynch, G. D. Myer, K. R. Ford, R. C. Gwin, and R. S. Heidt. "Multiple Risk Factors Related to Familial Predisposition to Anterior Cruciate Ligament Injury: Fraternal Twin Sisters with Anterior Cruciate Ligament Ruptures." British Journal of Sports Medicine 44, no. 12 (2010): 848–55. https://doi. org/10.1136/bjsm.2008.055798.

Hewett, Timothy E., Gregory D. Myer, Kevin R. Ford, Mark V. Paterno, and Carmen E. Quatman. "The Sequence of Prevention: A Systematic Approach to Prevent Anterior Cruciate Ligament Injury." Clinical Orthopaedics & Related Research 470, no. 10 (2012): 2930–40. https://doi.org/10.1007/s11999-012-2440-2.

Hewett, Timothy E., Gregory D. Myer, and Bohdanna T. Zazulak. "Hamstrings to Quadriceps Peak Torque Ratios Diverge between Sexes with Increasing Isokinetic Angular Velocity." Journal of Science and Medicine in Sport 11, no. 5 (2008): 452–59. https://doi.org/10.1016/j.jsams.2007.04.009.

Hewett, Timothy E., and Bohdanna T. Zazulak. "The Costs Associated with ACL Injury." In Understanding and Preventing Non-Contact ACL Injury, edited by Timothy E. Hewett, Sandra J. Schultz , and Letha Y. Griffin. Human Kinetics, 2007.

Hewett, Timothy E., and Bohdanna T. Zazulak. "Rehabilitation Considerations for the Female Athlete." In Physical Rehabilitation of the Injured Athlete 4th ED, edited by James Andrews, Gary Harrelson, and Kevin Wilk. Elvesier, 2012.

Hewett, Timothy E., and Bohdanna T. Zazulak. "Clinical Basis: Epidemiology, Risk Factors, Mechanisms of Injury, and Prevention of Ligament Injuries of the Knee." In The Knee Joint: Surgical Techniques and Strategies, edited by Michel Bonnin, Ned Annunziato Amendola, Johan Bellemans, Steven J. MacDonald, and Jacques Menetrey. Springer, 2012.

Hewett, Timothy E., Bohdanna T. Zazulak, Gregory D. Myer, Kevin R. Ford. "A Review of Electromyographic Activation Levels, Timing Differences, and Increased Anterior Cruciate Ligament Injury Incidence in Female Athletes." British Journal of Sports Medicine 39, no. 6 (2005): 347–50. https://doi.org/10.1136/bjsm.2005.018572.

Hewett, Timothy E., Bohdanna T. Zazulak, and Gregory D. Myer. "Theories on How Neuromuscular Interventions May Influence ACL Injury Rates: EMG activity, Muscle Firing Patterns, and Pre-Activation." In Understanding and Preventing Non-Contact ACL Injury, edited by Timothy E. Hewett, Sandra J. Schultz , and Letha Y. Griffin. Human Kinetics, 2007.

Hewett, Timothy E., Bohdanna T. Zazulak, and Gregory D. Myer. "Effects of the Menstrual Cycle on Anterior Cruciate Ligament Injury Risk: A Systematic Review." The American Journal of Sports Medicine 35, no. 4 (2007): 659–68. https://doi. org/10.1177/0363546506295699.

Hides, Julie, Stephen Wilson, Warren Stanton, Shaun McMahon, Heidi Keto, Katie McMahon, Martina Bryant, and Carolyn Richardson. "An MRI Investigation Into the Function of the Transversus Abdominis Muscle During 'Drawing-In' of the Abdominal Wall." Spine 31, no. 6 (2006). https://doi.org/10.1097/01. brs.0000202740.86338.df.

Hirshkowitz, Max, Kaitlyn Whiton, Steven M. Albert, Cathy Alessi, Oliviero Bruni, Lydia DonCarlos, Nancy Hazen, et al. "National Sleep Foundation's Sleep Time Duration Recommendations: Methodology and Results Summary." Sleep Health 1, no. 1 (2015): 40–43. https://doi.org/10.1016/j.sleh.2014.12.010.

Hodges, P. W., J. E. Butler, D. K. McKenzie, and S. C. Gandevia. "Contraction of the Human Diaphragm during Rapid Postural Adjustments." The Journal of Physiology 505, no. 2 (1997): 539–48. https://doi.org/10.1111/j.1469-7793.1997.539bb.x.

Hodges, P.W., A.E. Martin Eriksson, Debra Shirley, and Simon C Gandevia. "Intra-Abdominal Pressure Increases Stiffness of the Lumbar Spine." Journal of Biomechanics 38, no. 9 (2005): 1873–80. https://doi.org/10.1016/j.jbiomech.2004.08.016.

Hodges, P.W., and S.C. Gandevia. "Activation of the Human Diaphragm during a Repetitive Postural Task." The Journal of Physiology 522, no. 1 (2000): 165–75. https://doi.org/10.1111/j.1469-7793.2000. t01-1-00165.xm.

Hodges, P.W., and Simon C. Gandevia. "Changes in Intra-Abdominal Pressure during Postural and Respiratory Activation of the Human Diaphragm." Journal of Applied Physiology 89, no. 3 (2000): 967–76. https://doi.org/10.1152/jappl.2000.89.3.967.

Hodges, P.W., V. S. Gurfinkel, S. Brumagne, T. C. Smith, and P. C. Cordo. "Coexistence of Stability and Mobility in Postural

Control: Evidence from Postural Compensation for Respiration." Experimental Brain Research 144, no. 3 (2002): 293–302. https://doi.org/10.1007/s00221-002-1040-x.

Hodges, P.W, I. Heijnen, and S. C Gandevia. "Postural Activity of the Diaphragm Is Reduced in Humans When Respiratory Demand Increases." The Journal of Physiology 537, no. 3 (2001): 999–1008. https://doi.org/10.1113/jphysiol.2001.012648.

Hodges, P.W., R. Sapsford, and L.H.M. Pengel. "Postural and Respiratory Functions of the Pelvic Floor Muscles." Neurourology and Urodynamics 26, no. 3 (2007): 362–71. https://doi.org/10.1002/nau.20232.

Hodges, Paul W., and Carolyn A. Richardson. "Delayed Postural Contraction of Transversus Abdominis in Low Back Pain Associated with Movement of the Lower Limb." Journal of Spinal Disorders 11, no. 1 (1998). https://doi.org/10.1097/00002517-199802000-00008.

Hoffmann, Sven, Lea Teresa Jendreizik, Ulrich Ettinger, and Sylvain Laborde. "Keeping the Pace: The Effect of Slow-Paced Breathing on Error Monitoring." International Journal of Psychophysiology 146 (2019): 217–24. https://doi.org/10.1016/j.ijpsycho.2019.10.001.

Horsak, Brian, Rüdiger Wunsch, Philipp Bernhart, Anna-Maria Gorgas, Romana Bichler, and Kerstin Lampel. "Trunk Muscle Activation Levels during Eight Stabilization Exercises Used in the Functional Kinetics Concept: A Controlled Laboratory Study." Journal of Back and Musculoskeletal Rehabilitation 30, no. 3 (2017): 497–508. https://doi.org/10.3233/bmr-140259.

Hoy, Sara, Josefine Östh, Michaela Pascoe, Aaron Kandola, and Mats Hallgren. "Effects of Yoga-Based Interventions on Cognitive Function in Healthy Older Adults: A Systematic Review of Randomized Controlled Trials." Complementary Therapies in Medicine 58 (2021): 102690. https://doi.org/10.1016/j.ctim.2021.102690.

Hsu, Shih-Lin, Harumi Oda, Saya Shirahata, Mana Watanabe, and Makoto Sasaki. "Effects of Core Strength Training on Core

Stability." Journal of Physical Therapy Science 30, no. 8 (2018): 1014–18. https://doi.org/10.1589/jpts.30.1014.

Hunter, Sandra K. "The Relevance of Sex Differences in Performance Fatigability." Medicine & Science in Sports & Exercise 48, no. 11 (2016): 2247–56. https://doi.org/10.1249/mss.0000000000000928.

Hwang, Ui-jae, Min-seok Lee, Sung-hoon Jung, Sun-hee Ahn, and Oh-yun Kwon. "Effect of Pelvic Floor Electrical Stimulation on Diaphragm Excursion and Rib Cage Movement during Tidal and Forceful Breathing and Coughing in Women with Stress Urinary Incontinence." Medicine 100, no. 1 (2021). https://doi.org/10.1097/md.0000000000024158.

Imai, Atsushi, Koji Kaneoka, Yu Okubo, Itsuo Shiina, Masaki Tatsumura, Shigeki Izumi, and Hitoshi Shiraki. "Trunk Muscle Activity During Lumbar Stabilization Exercises on Both a Stable and Unstable Surface." Journal of Orthopaedic & Sports Physical Therapy 40, no. 6 (2010): 369–75. https://doi.org/10.2519/jospt.2010.3211.

Jang, Eun-Mi, Mi-Hyun Kim, and Jae-Seop Oh. "Effects of a Bridging Exercise with Hip Adduction on the EMG Activities of the Abdominal and Hip Extensor Muscles in Females." Journal of Physical Therapy Science 25, no. 9 (2013): 1147–49. https://doi.org/10.1589/jpts.25.1147.

Jeong, Jiyoung, Dai-Hyuk Choi, and Choongsoo S. Shin. "Core Strength Training Can Alter Neuromuscular and Biomechanical Risk Factors for Anterior Cruciate Ligament Injury." The American Journal of Sports Medicine 49, no. 1 (2021): 183–92. https://doi.org/10.1177/0363546520972990.

Josselyn, Sheena A., and Susumu Tonegawa. "Memory Engrams: Recalling the Past and Imagining the Future." Science 367, no. 6473 (2020). https://doi.org/10.1126/science.aaw4325.

Kajimura, Shogo, Naoki Masuda, Johnny King Lau, and Kou Murayama. "Focused Attention Meditation Changes the Boundary and Configuration of Functional Networks in the Brain." Scientific

Reports 10, no. 1 (2020). https://doi.org/10.1038/s41598-020-75396-9.

Katz, David L. "Plant-Based Diets for Reversing Disease and Saving the Planet: Past, Present, and Future." Advances in Nutrition 10, no. Supplement_4 (2019). https://doi.org/10.1093/advances/nmy124.

Kegel, Arnold H. "Progressive Resistance Exercise in the Functional Restoration of the Perineal Muscles." American Journal of Obstetrics and Gynecology 56, no. 2 (1948): 238–48. https://doi.org/10.1016/0002-9378(48)90266-x.

Khayambashi, Khalil, Navid Ghoddosi, Rachel K. Straub, and Christopher M. Powers. "Hip Muscle Strength Predicts Noncontact Anterior Cruciate Ligament Injury in Male and Female Athletes: A Prospective Study." The American Journal of Sports Medicine 44, no. 2 (2016): 355–61. https://doi.org/10.1177/0363546515616237.

Kibler, W Ben, Joel Press, and Aaron Sciascia. "The Role of Core Stability in Athletic Function." Sports Medicine 36, no. 3 (2006): 189–98. https://doi.org/10.2165/00007256-200636030-00001.

Kim, Chung Reen, Dae Kwon Park, Seok Tae Lee, and Ju Seok Ryu. "Electromyographic Changes in Trunk Muscles During Graded Lumbar Stabilization Exercises." PM&R 8, no. 10 (2016): 979–89. https://doi.org/10.1016/j.pmrj.2016.05.017.

Kim, Soo-Yong, Min-Hyeok Kang, Eui-Ryong Kim, In-Gui Jung, Eun-Young Seo, and Jae-seop Oh. "Comparison of EMG Activity on Abdominal Muscles during Plank Exercise with Unilateral and Bilateral Additional Isometric Hip Adduction." Journal of Electromyography and Kinesiology 30 (2016): 9–14. https://doi.org/10.1016/j.jelekin.2016.05.003.

Kolar, P., J. Sulc, M. Kyncl, J. Sanda, J. Neuwirth, A. V. Bokarius, J. Kriz, and A. Kobesova. "Stabilizing Function of the Diaphragm: Dynamic MRI and Synchronized Spirometric Assessment." Journal of Applied Physiology 109, no. 4 (2010): 1064–71. https://doi.org/10.1152/japplphysiol.01216.2009.

Kong, Yong-soo, Seol Park, Mi-Gyong Kweon, and Ji-won Park. "Change in Trunk Muscle Activities with Prone Bridge Exercise in Patients with Chronic Low Back Pain." Journal of Physical Therapy Science 28, no. 1 (2016): 264–68. https://doi.org/10.1589/jpts.28.264.

Krishnan, Bindu, Rama Krishna Sanjeev, R.G Latti. "Quality of Sleep Among Bedtime Smartphone Users." International Journal of Preventive Medicine 11, no. 1 (2020):114. https://doi.org/10.4103/ijpvm.ijpvm_266_19.

Krishnan, Dolly. "Orchestration of Dreams: a Possible Tool for Enhancement of Mental Productivity and Efficiency." Sleep and Biological Rhythms (2021): 1-7. https://doi.org/10.1007/s41105-021-00313-0.

Kruk, Joanna, Katarzyna Kotarska, and Basil H. Aboul-Enein. "Physical Exercise and Catecholamines Response: Benefits and Health Risk: Possible Mechanisms." Free Radical Research 54, no. 2-3 (2020): 105–25. https://doi.org/10.1080/10715762.2020.1726343.

Kuether, Justin, Anne Moore, Joseph Kahan, Joseph Martucci, Tara Messina, Roland Perreault, Robert Sembler, et al. "Telerehabilitation for Total Hip and Knee Arthroplasty Patients: A Pilot Series with High Patient Satisfaction." HSS Journal ® 15, no. 3 (2019): 221–25. https://doi.org/10.1007/s11420-019-09715-

Leathers, Michael, Alexa Merz, Jeffrey Wong, Trevor Scott, Jeffrey Wang, and Sharon Hame. "Trends and Demographics in Anterior Cruciate Ligament Reconstruction in the United States." Journal of Knee Surgery 28, no. 05 (2015): 390–94. https://doi.org/10.1055/s-0035-1544193.

Lee, Angela S., Jacek Cholewicki, N. Peter Reeves, Bohdanna T. Zazulak, and Lawrence W. Mysliwiec. "Comparison of Trunk Proprioception Between Patients With Low Back Pain and Healthy Controls." Archives of Physical Medicine and Rehabilitation 91, no. 9 (2010): 1327–31. https://doi.org/10.1016/j.apmr.2010.06.004.

Lee, Darrin J., Edwin Kulubya, Philippe Goldin, Amir Goodarzi, and Fady Girgis. "Review of the Neural Oscillations Underlying Meditation." Frontiers in Neuroscience 12 (2018). https://doi.org/10.3389/fnins.2018.00178.

Lee, Su-Kyoung. "The Effects of Abdominal Drawing-in Maneuver during Stair Climbing on Muscle Activities of the Trunk and Legs." Journal of Exercise Rehabilitation 15, no. 2 (2019): 224–28. https://doi.org/10.12965/jer.1938056.028.

Leetun, Darin T., Mary Lloyd Ireland, John D. Willson, Bryon T. Ballantyne, and Irene McClay Davis. "Core Stability Measures as Risk Factors for Lower Extremity Injury in Athletes." Medicine & Science in Sports & Exercise 36, no. 6 (2004): 926–34. https://doi.org/10.1249/01.mss.0000128145.75199.c3.

Lewis, Cara L., Hanna D. Foley, Theresa S. Lee, and Justin W. Berry. "Hip-Muscle Activity in Men and Women During Resisted Side Stepping With Different Band Positions." Journal of Athletic Training 53, no. 11 (2018): 1071–81. https://doi.org/10.4085/1062-6050-46-16.

Levine, Glenn N., Beth E. Cohen, Yvonne Commodore-Mensah, Julie Fleury, Jeff C. Huffman, Umair Khalid, Darwin R. Labarthe, et al. "Psychological Health, Well-Being, and the Mind-Heart-Body Connection: A Scientific Statement From the American Heart Association." Circulation 143, no. 10 (2021). https://doi.org/10.1161/cir.0000000000000947.

L'Hermette, Maxime, Ingrid Castres, Jeremy Coquart, Montassar Tabben, Nihel Ghoul, Bernard Andrieu, and Claire Tourny. "Cold Water Immersion After a Handball Training Session: The Relationship Between Physical Data and Sensorial Experience." Frontiers in Sports and Active Living 2 (2020). https://doi.org/10.3389/fspor.2020.581705.

Lohani, Monika, Kara McElvaine, Brennan Payne, Kate Mitcheom, and Willoughby Britton. "A Longitudinal Training Study to Delineate the Specific Causal Effects of Open Monitoring Versus Focused Attention Techniques on Emotional Health." Complementary Therapies in Medicine 53 (2020): 102525. https://doi.org/10.1016/j.ctim.2020.102525.

Lopes, Thiago Jambo, Milena Simic, Gregory D. Myer, Kevin R. Ford, Timothy E. Hewett, and Evangelos Pappas. "The Effects of Injury Prevention Programs on the Biomechanics of Landing Tasks: A Systematic Review With Meta-Analysis." The American Journal of Sports Medicine 46, no. 6 (2017): 1492–99. https://doi.org/10.1177/0363546517716930.

Macdonald, Ian, John S. Rubin, Ed Blake, Shashi Hirani, and Ruth Epstein. "An Investigation of Abdominal Muscle Recruitment for Sustained Phonation in 25 Healthy Singers." Journal of Voice 26, no. 6 (2012). https://doi.org/10.1016/j.jvoice.2012.04.006.

Madokoro, Sachiko, Masami Yokogawa, and Hiroichi Miaki. "Effect of the Abdominal Draw-In Maneuver and Bracing on Abdominal Muscle Thickness and the Associated Subjective Difficulty in Healthy Individuals." Healthcare 8, no. 4 (2020): 496. https://doi.org/10.3390/healthcare8040496.

Magnusson, Karin, Aleksandra Turkiewicz, Velocity Hughes, Richard Frobell, Martin Englund. "High genetic contribution to anterior cruciate ligament rupture: Heritability ~69." British Journal of Sports Medicine (2020): https://doi.org/10.1136/bjsports-2020-102392.

Mäkinen, Tiina M., Matti Mäntysaari, Tiina Pääkkönen, Jari Jokelainen, Lawrence A. Palinkas, Juhani Hassi, Juhani Leppäluoto, Kari Tahvanainen, and Hannu Rintamäki. "Autonomic Nervous Function During Whole-Body Cold Exposure Before and After Cold Acclimation." Aviation, Space, and Environmental Medicine 79, no. 9 (2008): 875–82. https://doi.org/10.3357/asem.2235.2008.

Massery, M., M. Hagins, R. Stafford, V. Moerchen, and P. W. Hodges. "Effect of Airway Control by Glottal Structures on Postural Stability." Journal of Applied Physiology 115, no. 4 (2013): 483–90. https://doi.org/10.1152/japplphysiol.01226.2012.

Matusheski, Nathan V., Aoife Caffrey, Lars Christensen, Simon Mezgec, Shelini Surendran, Mads F. Hjorth, Helene McNulty, et al. "Diets, Nutrients, Genes and the Microbiome: Recent Advances in Personalised Nutrition." British Journal of Nutrition (2021, 1–9. https://doi.org/10.1017/s0007114521000374.

McGill, Stuart M., Aaron Childs, and Craig Liebenson. "Endurance Times for Low Back Stabilization Exercises: Clinical Targets for Testing and Training from a Normal Database." Archives of Physical Medicine and Rehabilitation 80, no. 8 (1999): 941–44. https://doi.org/10.1016/s0003-9993(99)90087-4.

McPherson, April L., Julian A. Feller, Timothy E. Hewett, and Kate E. Webster. "Smaller Change in Psychological Readiness to Return to Sport Is Associated With Second Anterior Cruciate Ligament Injury Among Younger Patients." The American Journal of Sports Medicine 47, no. 5 (2019): 1209–15. https://doi.org/10.1177/0363546519825499.

McPherson, April L., Julian A. Feller, Timothy E. Hewett, and Kate E. Webster. "Psychological Readiness to Return to Sport Is Associated With Second Anterior Cruciate Ligament Injuries." The American Journal of Sports Medicine 47, no. 4 (2019): 857–62. https://doi.org/10.1177/0363546518825258.

Medvecky, Michael J., Bohdanna T. Zazulak, and Timothy E. Hewett. "A Multidisciplinary Approach to the Evaluation, Reconstruction and Rehabilitation of the Multi-Ligament Injured Athlete." Sports Medicine 37, no. 2 (2007): 169–87. https://doi.org/10.2165/00007256-200737020-00005.

Meehan, William P., Marc G. Weisskopf, Supriya Krishnan, Caitlin McCracken, Ross Zafonte, Herman A. Taylor, Aaron Baggish, Alvaro Pascual-Leone, Lee M. Nadler, and Frank E. Speizer. "Relation of Anterior Cruciate Ligament Tears to Potential Chronic Cardiovascular diseases." The American Journal of Cardiology vol. 122,11 (2018): 1879-1884. https://doi.org/10.1016/j.amjcard.2018.08.030.

Meier, Maria, Eva Unternaehrer, Stephanie J. Dimitroff, Annika B. Benz, Ulrike U. Bentele, Sabine M. Schorpp, Maya Wenzel, and Jens C. Pruessner. "Standardized Massage Interventions as Protocols for the Induction of Psychophysiological Relaxation in the Laboratory: a Block Randomized, Controlled Trial." Scientific Reports 10, no. 1 (2020). https://doi.org/10.1038/s41598-020-71173-w.

Meredith, Sean J., Thomas Rauer, Terese L. Chmielewski, Christian Fink, Theresa Diermeier, Benjamin B. Rothrauff, Eleonor Svantesson, et al. "Return to Sport after Anterior Cruciate Ligament Injury: Panther Symposium ACL Injury Return to Sport Consensus Group." Knee Surgery, Sports Traumatology, Arthroscopy 28, no. 8 (2020): 2403–14. https://doi.org/10.1007/s00167-020-06009-1.

Miry, Omid, Jie Li, and Lu Chen. "The Quest for the Hippocampal Memory Engram: From Theories to Experimental Evidence." Frontiers in Behavioral Neuroscience 14 (2021). https://doi.org/10.3389/fnbeh.2020.632019.

Mok, Nicola W., Ella W. Yeung, Jeran C. Cho, Samson C. Hui, Kimee C. Liu, and Coleman H. Pang. "Core Muscle Activity during Suspension Exercises." Journal of Science and Medicine in Sport 18, no. 2 (2015): 189–94. https://doi.org/10.1016/j.jsams.2014.01.002.

Moser, Helene, Monika Leitner, Jean-Pierre Baeyens, and Lorenz Radlinger. "Pelvic Floor Muscle Activity during Impact Activities in Continent and Incontinent Women: a Systematic Review." International Urogynecology Journal 29, no. 2 (2018): 179–96. https://doi.org/10.1007/s00192-017-3441-1.

Myer, Gregory D., Kevin R. Ford, Scott G. McLean, and Timothy E. Hewett. "The Effects of Plyometric versus Dynamic Stabilization and Balance Training on Lower Extremity Biomechanics." The American Journal of Sports Medicine 34, no. 3 (2006): 445–55. https://doi.org/10.1177/0363546505281241.

Nagelli, Christopher V., Kate E. Webster, Stephanie Di Stasi, Samuel C. Wordeman, and Timothy E. Hewett. "The Association of Psychological Readiness to Return to Sport after Anterior Cruciate Ligament Reconstruction and Hip and Knee Landing Kinematics." Clinical Biomechanics 68 (2019): 104–8. https://doi.org/10.1016/j.clinbiomech.2019.05.031.

Nascimento, Simone S., Larissa R. Oliveira, and Josimari M. DeSantana. "Correlations between Brain Changes and Pain Management after Cognitive and Meditative Therapies: A Systematic Review of Neuroimaging Studies." Complementary Therapies in Medicine 39 (2018): 137–45. https://doi.org/10.1016/j.ctim.2018.06.006.

Ni, Meng, Kiersten Mooney, Kysha Harriell, Anoop Balachandran, and Joseph Signorile. "Core Muscle Function during Specific Yoga Poses." Complementary Therapies in Medicine 22, no. 2 (2014): 235–43. https://doi.org/10.1016/j.ctim.2014.01.007.

Okubo, Yu, Koji Kaneoka, Atsushi Imai, Itsuo Shiina, Masaki Tatsumura, Shigeki Izumi, and Shumpei Miyakawa. "Electromyographic Analysis of Transversus Abdominis and Lumbar Multifidus Using Wire Electrodes During Lumbar Stabilization Exercises." Journal of Orthopaedic & Sports Physical Therapy 40, no. 11 (2010): 743–50. https://doi.org/10.2519/jospt.2010.3192.

Oliva-Lozano, José M., and José M. Muyor. "Core Muscle Activity during Physical Fitness Exercises: A Systematic Review." International Journal of Environmental Research and Public Health 17, no. 12 (2020): 4306. https://doi.org/10.3390/ijerph17124306.

Oliver, Gretchen D., Jessica K. Washington, Jeff W. Barfield, Sarah S. Gascon, and Gabrielle Gilmer. "Quantitative Analysis of Proximal and Distal Kinetic Chain Musculature During Dynamic Exercises." Journal of Strength and Conditioning Research 32, no. 6 (2018): 1545–53. https://doi.org/10.1519/jsc.0000000000002036.

Oman, Doug, Jill E. Bormann, and Jim J. Kane. "Mantram Repetition as a Portable Mindfulness Practice: Applications During the COVID-19 Pandemic." Mindfulness, 2020. https://doi.org/10.1007/s12671-020-01545-w.

Panhan, Ana C., Mauro Gonçalves, Giovana D. Eltz, Marina M. Villalba, Adalgiso C. Cardozo, and Fausto Bérzin. "Neuromuscular Efficiency of the Multifidus Muscle in Pilates Practitioners and Non-Practitioners." Complementary Therapies in Medicine 40 (2018): 61–63. https://doi.org/10.1016/j.ctim.2018.07.014.

Pappas, Evangelos, Bohdanna T. Zazulak, and Lee D. Katz. "Enchondroma in a Running Athlete With Persistent Mid-Thigh Pain." Journal of Orthopaedic & Sports Physical Therapy 40, no. 2 (2010): 121–21. https://doi.org/10.2519/jospt.2010.0403.

Pappas, Evangelos, Bohdanna T. Zazulak, Ellen E. Yard, and Timothy E. Hewett. "The Epidemiology of Pediatric Basketball Injuries

Presenting to US Emergency Departments: 2000-2006." Sports Health: A Multidisciplinary Approach 3, no. 4 (2011): 331–35. https://doi.org/10.1177/1941738111409861.

Park, Denise C, and Gérard N Bischof. "The aging mind: neuroplasticity in response to cognitive training." Dialogues in clinical neuroscience 15, no. 1 (2013): 109-19. https://doi.org/10.31887/DCNS.2013.15.1/dpark.

Park, Hankyu, and Dongwook Han. "The Effect of the Correlation between the Contraction of the Pelvic Floor Muscles and Diaphragmatic Motion during Breathing." Journal of Physical Therapy Science 27, no. 7 (2015): 2113–15. https://doi.org/10.1589/jpts.27.2113.

Pena, Caroline C., Kari Bø, Aura M. Ossa, Ana C. Fernandes, Devechio N. Aleixo, Flávia M. Oliveira, and Cristine H. Ferreira. "Are Visual Inspection and Digital Palpation Reliable Methods to Assess Ability to Perform a Pelvic Floor Muscle Contraction? An Intra-Rater Study." Neurourology and Urodynamics 40, no. 2 (2021): 680–87. https://doi.org/10.1002/nau.24609.

Phillips, Edward M., Elizabeth P. Frates, and David J. Park. "Lifestyle Medicine." Physical Medicine and Rehabilitation Clinics of North America 31, no. 4 (2020): 515–26. https://doi.org/10.1016/j.pmr.2020.07.006.

Plisky, Phillip J., Mitchell J. Rauh, Thomas W. Kaminski, and Frank B. Underwood. "Star Excursion Balance Test as a Predictor of Lower Extremity Injury in High School Basketball Players." Journal of Orthopaedic & Sports Physical Therapy 36, no. 12 (2006): 911–19. https://doi.org/10.2519/jospt.2006.2244.

Pogetti, Lívia Silveira, Theresa Helissa Nakagawa, Giovanna Prado Conteçote, and Paula Rezende Camargo. "Core Stability, Shoulder Peak Torque and Function in Throwing Athletes with and without Shoulder Pain." Physical Therapy in Sport 34 (2018): 36–42. https://doi.org/10.1016/j.ptsp.2018.08.008.

Proske, Uwe. "Exercise, Fatigue and Proprioception: a Retrospective." Experimental Brain Research 237, no. 10 (2019): 2447–59. https://doi.org/10.1007/s00221-019-05634-8.

Radebold, Andrea, Jacek Cholewicki, Gert K. Polzhofer, and Hunter S. Greene. "Impaired Postural Control of the Lumbar Spine Is Associated With Delayed Muscle Response Times in Patients With Chronic Idiopathic Low Back Pain." Spine 26, no. 7 (2001): 724–30. https://doi.org/10.1097/00007632-200104010-00004.

Peter Reeves, N., Kumpati S. Narendra, and Jacek Cholewicki. "Spine Stability: The Six Blind Men and the Elephant." Clinical Biomechanics 22, no. 3 (2007): 266–74. https://doi.org/10.1016/j.clinbiomech.2006.11.011.

Richardson, Eleanor, Jeremy S Lewis, Jo Gibson, Chris Morgan, Mark Halaki, Karen Ginn, and Gillian Yeowell. "Role of the Kinetic Chain in Shoulder Rehabilitation: Does Incorporating the Trunk and Lower Limb into Shoulder Exercise Regimes Influence Shoulder Muscle Recruitment Patterns? Systematic Review of Electromyography Studies." BMJ Open Sport & Exercise Medicine 6, no. 1 (2020). https://doi.org/10.1136/bmjsem-2019-000683.

Riebl, Shaun K., and Brenda M. Davy. "The Hydration Equation." ACSM'S Health & Fitness Journal 17, no. 6 (2013): 21–28. https://doi.org/10.1249/fit.0b013e3182a9570f.

Rodríguez-López, Elena Sonsoles, Sofía Olivia Calvo-Moreno, Ángel Basas-García, Fernando Gutierrez-Ortega, Jesús Guodemar-Pérez, and María Barbaño Acevedo-Gómez. "Prevalence of Urinary Incontinence among Elite Athletes of Both Sexes." Journal of Science and Medicine in Sport 24, no. 4 (2021): 338–44. https://doi.org/10.1016/j.jsams.2020.09.017.

Rudavsky, Aliza, and Tricia Turner. "Novel Insight into the Coordination between Pelvic Floor Muscles and the Glottis through Ultrasound Imaging: a Pilot Study." International Urogynecology Journal 31, no. 12 (2020): 2645–52. https://doi.org/10.1007/s00192-020-04461-8.

Sasaki, Shizuka, Eiichi Tsuda, Yuji Yamamoto, Shugo Maeda, Yuka Kimura, Yuki Fujita, and Yasuyuki Ishibashi. "Core-Muscle Training and Neuromuscular Control of the Lower Limb and Trunk." Journal of Athletic Training 54, no. 9 (2019): 959–69. https://doi.org/10.4085/1062-6050-113-17.

Schilaty, Nathan D., Christopher Nagelli, and Timothy E. Hewett. "Use of Objective Neurocognitive Measures to Assess the Psychological States That Influence Return to Sport Following Injury." Sports Medicine 46, no. 3 (2016): 299–303. https://doi.org/10.1007/s40279-015-0435-3.

Schwalm, Fábio Duarte, Rafaela Brugalli Zandavalli, Eno Dias de Castro Filho, and Giancarlo Lucchetti. "Is There a Relationship between Spirituality/Religiosity and Resilience? A Systematic Review and Meta-Analysis of Observational Studies." Journal of Health Psychology, 2021, 135910532098453. https://doi.org/10.1177/1359105320984537.

Selkow, Noelle M., Molly R. Eck, and Stephen Rivas. "Transversus Abdominis Activation and Timing Improves Following Core Stability Training: A Randomized Trial." International Journal of Sports Physical Therapy 12, no. 7 (2017): 1048–56. https://doi.org/10.26603/ijspt20171048.

Sheehan, Connor M, Stephen E Frochen, Katrina M Walsemann, and Jennifer A Ailshire. "Are U.S. Adults Reporting Less Sleep?: Findings from Sleep Duration Trends in the National Health Interview Survey, 2004–2017." Sleep 42, no. 2 (2019). https://doi.org/10.1093/sleep/zsy221.

Smith, Craig A., Nicole J. Chimera, and Meghan Warren. "Association of Y Balance Test Reach Asymmetry and Injury in Division I Athletes." Medicine & Science in Sports & Exercise 47, no. 1 (2015): 136–41. https://doi.org/10.1249/mss.0000000000000380.

Smith, Helen C., Pamela Vacek, Robert J. Johnson, James R. Slauterbeck, Javad Hashemi, Sandra Shultz, and Bruce D. Beynnon. "Risk Factors for Anterior Cruciate Ligament Injury." Sports Health: A Multidisciplinary Approach 4, no. 2 (2012): 155–61. https://doi.org/10.1177/1941738111428282.

Snarr, Ronald L., and Michael R. Esco. "Electromyographical Comparison of Plank Variations Performed With and Without Instability Devices." Journal of Strength and Conditioning Research 28, no. 11 (2014): 3298–3305. https://doi.org/10.1519/jsc.0000000000000521.

Snarr, Ronald L., Ashleigh V. Hallmark, Brett S. Nickerson, and Michael R. Esco. "Electromyographical Comparison of Pike Variations Performed With and Without Instability Devices." Journal of Strength and Conditioning Research 30, no. 12 (2016): 3436–42. https://doi.org/10.1519/jsc.0000000000001436.

Song, Qipeng, Li Li, Cui Zhang Wei Sun, and Dewei Mao. "Long-term Tai Chi practitioners have superior body stability under dual task condition during stair ascent." Gait Posture (2018):124-129. https://doi.org/10.1016/j.gaitpost.2018.08.008.

Stookey, Jodi D., Stavros A. Kavouras, HyunGyu Suh, and Florian Lang. "Underhydration Is Associated with Obesity, Chronic Diseases, and Death Within 3 to 6 Years in the U.S. Population Aged 51–70 Years." Nutrients 12, no. 4 (2020): 905. https://doi.org/10.3390/nu12040905.

Sugimoto, Dai, Carl G. Mattacola, Heather M. Bush, Staci M. Thomas, Kim D. Foss, Gregory D. Myer, and Timothy E. Hewett. "Preventive Neuromuscular Training for Young Female Athletes: Comparison of Coach and Athlete Compliance Rates." Journal of Athletic Training 52, no. 1 (2017): 58–64. https://doi.org/10.4085/1062-6050-51.12.20.

Sugimoto, Dai, Gregory D. Myer, Heather M. Bush, and Timothy E. Hewett. "Effects of Compliance on Trunk and Hip Integrative Neuromuscular Training on Hip Abductor Strength in Female Athletes." Journal of Strength and Conditioning Research 28, no. 5 (2014): 1187–94. https://doi.org/10.1097/jsc.0000000000000228.

Talasz, Helena, Christian Kremser, Markus Kofler, Elisabeth Kalchschmid, Monika Lechleitner, and Ansgar Rudisch. "Phase-Locked Parallel Movement of Diaphragm and Pelvic Floor during Breathing and Coughing—a Dynamic MRI Investigation in Healthy Females." International Urogynecology Journal 22, no. 1 (2011): 61–68. https://doi.org/10.1007/s00192-010-1240-z.

Talasz, Helena, Markus Kofler, Elisabeth Kalchschmid, Michael Pretterklieber, and Monika Lechleitner. "Breathing with the Pelvic Floor? Correlation of Pelvic Floor Muscle Function

and Expiratory Flows in Healthy Young Nulliparous Women."
International Urogynecology Journal 21, no. 4 (2010): 475–81.
https://doi.org/10.1007/s00192-009-1060-1.

Tiwari, Reena, Ravindra Kumar, Sujata Malik, Tilak Raj, and Punit
Kumar. "Analysis of Heart Rate Variability and Implication
of Different Factors on Heart Rate Variability." Current
Cardiology Reviews 16 (2020). https://doi.org/10.2174/157340
3x16999201231203854.

Trivedi, GunjanY, Vidhi Patel, MeghalH Shah, MeghanaJ Dhok, and
Kunal Bhoyania. "Comparative Study of the Impact of Active
Meditation Protocol and Silence Meditation on Heart Rate
Variability and Mood in Women." International Journal of Yoga
13, no. 3 (2020): 255. https://doi.org/10.4103/ijoy.ijoy_18_20.

Troyer, André De, and Theodore A. Wilson. "Action of the Diaphragm
on the Rib Cage." Journal of Applied Physiology 121, no. 2 (2016):
391–400. https://doi.org/10.1152/japplphysiol.00268.2016.

Tymofiyeva, Olga, and Robert Gaschler. "Training-Induced Neural
Plasticity in Youth: A Systematic Review of Structural and
Functional MRI Studies." Frontiers in Human Neuroscience 14
(2021). https://doi.org/10.3389/fnhum.2020.497245.

United States Bone and Joint Initiative: The Burden of Musculoskeletal
Diseases in the United States (BMUS), Third Edition, 2014.
Rosemont, IL. ISBN: 978-0-9963091-0-3. 2018. United States
Bone and Joint Initiative.

Verkhoshansky, Y. "Are depth jumps useful?" Soviet Sport Review no. 3
(1968): 75-78. Google Scholar.

Vesentini, Giovana, Regina El Dib, Leonardo Augusto Righesso,
Fernanda Piculo, Gabriela Marini, Guilherme Augusto Ferraz,
Iracema de Calderon, Angélica Mércia Barbosa, and Marilza Vieira
Rudge. "Pelvic Floor and Abdominal Muscle Cocontraction in
Women with and without Pelvic Floor Dysfunction: a Systematic
Review and Meta-Analysis." Clinics 74 (2019). https://doi.
org/10.6061/clinics/2019/e1319.

Vickhoff, Björn, Helge Malmgren, Rickard Åström, Gunnar Nyberg, Seth-Reino Ekström, Mathias Engwall, Johan Snygg, Michael Nilsson, and Rebecka Jörnsten. "Music Structure Determines Heart Rate Variability of Singers." Frontiers in Psychology 4 (2013). https://doi.org/10.3389/fpsyg.2013.00334.

Vodovotz, Yoram, Neal Barnard, Frank B. Hu, John Jakicic, Liana Lianov, David Loveland, Daniel Buysse, et al. "Prioritized Research for the Prevention, Treatment, and Reversal of Chronic Disease: Recommendations From the Lifestyle Medicine Research Summit." Frontiers in Medicine 7 (2020). https://doi.org/10.3389/fmed.2020.585744.

Wagner, Heiko, Ulrich Rehmes, Daniel Kohle, and Christian Puta. "Laughing: A Demanding Exercise for Trunk Muscles." Journal of Motor Behavior 46, no. 1 (2014): 33–37. https://doi.org/10.1080/00222895.2013.844091.

Walton, Lori Maria, Veena Raigangar, Mini Sara Abraham, Cherisse Buddy, Magaly Hernandez, Gretchen Krivak, and Rose Caceras. "Effects of an 8-Week Pelvic Core Stability and Nutrition Community Programme on Maternal Health Outcomes." Physiotherapy Research International 24, no. 4 (2019). https://doi.org/10.1002/pri.1780.

Wang, Chunguang, Hao Li, Kang Chen, Bing Wu, and Haifeng Liu. "Association of Polymorphisms rs1800012 in COL1A1 with Sports-Related Tendon and Ligament Injuries: a Meta-Analysis." Oncotarget 8, no. 16 (2017): 27627–34. https://doi.org/10.18632/oncotarget.15271.

Webster, Kate E., April L. McPherson, Timothy E. Hewett, and Julian A. Feller. "Factors Associated With a Return to Preinjury Level of Sport Performance After Anterior Cruciate Ligament Reconstruction Surgery." The American Journal of Sports Medicine 47, no. 11 (2019): 2557–62. https://doi.org/10.1177/0363546519865537.

Wilkerson, Gary B., Jessica L. Giles, and Dustin K. Seibel. "Prediction of Core and Lower Extremity Strains and Sprains in Collegiate Football Players: A Preliminary Study." Journal of Athletic

Training 47, no. 3 (2012): 264–72. https://doi.org/10.4085/1062-6050-47.3.17.

Wilkerson, Gary B., and Marisa A. Colston. "A Refined Prediction Model for Core and Lower Extremity Sprains and Strains Among Collegiate Football Players." Journal of Athletic Training 50, no. 6 (2015): 643–50. https://doi.org/10.4085/1062-6050-50.2.04.

Willson, John D., Christopher P. Dougherty, Mary Lloyd Ireland, and Irene McClay Davis. "Core Stability and Its Relationship to Lower Extremity Function and Injury." Journal of the American Academy of Orthopaedic Surgeons 13, no. 5 (2005): 316–25. https://doi.org/10.5435/00124635-200509000-00005.

Wilt, Fred. "Plyometrics: What is it and how it works." Modern Athlete and Coach, 16 (1978): 9–12. Google Scholar.

Yun, Byeong-Gwon, Seung-Joo Lee, Hyun-Jeong So, and Won-Seob Shin. "Changes in Muscle Activity of the Abdominal Muscles According to Exercise Method and Speed during Dead Bug Exercise." Physical Therapy Rehabilitation Science 6, no. 1 (2017): 1–6. https://doi.org/10.14474/ptrs.2017.6.1.1.

Zachovajeviene, B., L. Siupsinskas, P. Zachovajevas, Z. Venclovas, and D. Milonas. "Effect of Diaphragm and Abdominal Muscle Training on Pelvic Floor Strength and Endurance: Results of a Prospective Randomized Trial." Scientific Reports 9, no. 1 (2019). https://doi.org/10.1038/s41598-019-55724-4.

Zazulak, Bohdanna T., Timothy E. Hewett, N. Peter Reeves, Barry Goldberg, and Jacek Cholewicki. "Deficits in Neuromuscular Control of the Trunk Predict Knee Injury Risk." The American Journal of Sports Medicine 35, no. 7 (2007): 1123–30. https://doi.org/10.1177/0363546507301585.

Zazulak, Bohdanna T., Timothy E. Hewett, N. Peter Reeves, Barry Goldberg, and Jacek Cholewicki. "The Effects of Core Proprioception on Knee Injury." The American Journal of Sports Medicine 35, no. 3 (2007): 368–73. https://doi.org/10.1177/0363546506297909.

Zazulak, Bohdanna T. and Michael J. Medvecky. "Trunk Stability for Injury Prevention: The Core of Evidence." Connecticut Medicine 83, no. 9 (2019): 443-450. http://ctmed.csms.org/publication/?i=623737&p=13&pp=1&view=issueViewer.

Zazulak, Bohdanna T., Mark Paterno, Gregory D Myer, William A Romani, and Timothy E Hewett. "The Effects of the Menstrual Cycle on Anterior Knee Laxity." Sports Medicine 36, no. 10 (2006): 847–62. https://doi.org/10.2165/00007256-200636100-00004.

Zazulak, Bohdanna T., Patricia L. Ponce, Stephen J. Straub, Michael J. Medvecky, Lori Avedisian, and Timothy E. Hewett. "Gender Comparison of Hip Muscle Activity During Single-Leg Landing." Journal of Orthopaedic & Sports Physical Therapy 35, no. 5 (2005): 292–99. https://doi.org/10.2519/jospt.2005.35.5.292.

Zazulak, Bohdanna T., Jacek Cholewicki, and Peter N. Reeves. "Neuromuscular Control of Trunk Stability: Clinical Implications for Sports Injury Prevention." Journal of the American Academy of Orthopaedic Surgeons 16, no. 8 (2008): 497–505. https://doi.org/10.5435/00124635-200808000-00011.

CONNECT WITH
DR. BOHDANNA ZAZULAK

Sign up for Bohdanna's newsletter at
www.doczaz.com/newsletter

To find out more information visit her website:
www.doczaz.com

BOOK DISCOUNTS AND
SPECIAL DEALS

Sign up for free to get discounts and special deals
on our bestselling books at
www.TCKpublishing.com/bookdeals

Made in the USA
Coppell, TX
26 November 2022

87111821R00156